Harald-Robert Bruch

Local regional Electro-hyperthermia in patients with liver metastases from colorectal carcinoma: A case control study in three ambulatory oncological practices in Germany

SCIENTIA NOVA
Das interdisziplinäre Wissenschaftsmagazin
Sonderdruck 2/2014

Institut für Akademische Zusammenarbeit
Institute for Academic Cooperation

Marosi Verlag

Bibliographische Information der Deutschen Nationalbibliothek
Die Deutsche Nationalbibliothek verzeichnet diese Publikation in der Deutschen Nationalbibliographie. Detaillierte bibliographische Daten sind im Internet über http://dnb.d-nb.de abrufbar.

Prof. Dr. med. Harald-Robert Bruch, M.Sc., Ph.D.
Onkologie Rheinland, Praxiskooperation Bonn-Euskirchen-Rheinbach
für Blut- und Krebserkrankungen
Europaring 42, D-53123 Bonn
bonner-onkologen@t-online.de
www.onkologie-rheinland.de

© 2014 Marosi Verlag, Ludwigshafen am Rhein
marosiverlag@gmx.de &
Institut für Akademische Zusammenarbeit
Institute for Academic Cooperation
Tonhallenstraße 19, D-47051 Duisburg

Druck: Books on Demand GmbH, Norderstedt
Printed in Germany 2014

ISBN 978-3-945636-02-2
ISSN 1861-4043

Herausgeber	Institut für Akademische Zusammenarbeit Institute for Academic Cooperation Tonhallenstraße 19, D-47051 Duisburg Telefon +49 203 9413091 Telefax +49 203 9413092
Redaktionsleitung	Rechtsanwalt Dr. iur. JUDr. Klaus U. Groth (V.i.S.d.P.) Dr. oec. Rainer Schreiber (V.i.S.d.P.)
Ausführende Redakteurin/Verlag	Dr. phil. Silvia Marosi, Marosi Verlag, Ludwigshafen
Beirat	Prof. Dr. Jakov Beltschikov †, Riga Prof. Dr. Anatolij Chujkin, Königsberg Rechtsanwalt Dr. Adrian Hollaender, Wien Prof. Dr. Hans Klecatsky, Bundesjustizminister a.D., Innsbruck Dipl.-Kfm. Dr. Klaus Orth, M.A., Düsseldorf Prof. Dr. Pichan Sopikorn, Bangkok Prof. Dr. Chrysant von Sturm zu Vehlingen, St. Gallen

Contents

LIST OF ABBREVIATIONS

5-FU	5-Fluorouracil
A	Doxorubicin
AC	Alternating Current
ATP	Adenosine-5′-triphosphate
BCNU	Bis-chloroethylnitrosourea (Carmustine)
BNHO	Association of Haematologists and Oncologists in Germany
Carbo	Carboplatin
CDDP	Cisplatin
cem	cumulative equivalent minutes
CR	Complete remission
CT	Chemotherapy
CTL	Cytotoxic T Lymphocytes
DFS	Disease free survival
DNA	Deoxyribonucleic acid
Dr.	Doctor
DC	Dendritic cell
E	Etoposide
Gy	Gray
Hep G2	Liver hepatocellular cell line
HIP	Hyperthermal isolated organ perfusion
HIPEC	Hyperthermal intraperitoneal chemotherapy
HMGB1	High-Mobility-Group Protein B1
Hsp	Heat shock protein
HT	Hyperthermia
HT29	Human colon adenocarcinoma grade II cell line
I	Ifosfamid
i.p.	intraperitoneal
IFO	Ifosfamide
IHT	Interstitial hyperthermia
LPFS	local progression free survival
LRHT	Local regional hyperthermia
MBA	Master of Business Administration
med.	Medicine

MHC	Major histocompatibility complex
MHz	Megahertz
MMC	Mitomycin C
NCI	National Cancer Institute
NK-cell	Natural killer cell
°C	Degree Celsius
OS	overall survival
PBHT	Partial body hyperthermia
PFS	Progression Free Survival
Ph.D.	Doctor of Philosophy
PI	Principal Investigator
PR	Partial remission
Prof.	Professor
RF	Radiofrequency
RHT	Regional hyperthermia
RT	Radiotherapy
S-Phase	Synthesis phase of cell cycle
TID	Thermal isodose TID concept
VA	Voltampere
VP16	Etoposide
W	Watt
WBH	Whole body hyperthermia
WBH	Whole body hyperthermia

1. Introduction: Hyperthermia as an Oncological Therapy Concept

The effect of conventional cytotoxic therapy procedures in the area of tumour therapy such as drug therapy, chemotherapy, and radiotherapy can be reinforced through heat.

Along with the direct cytotoxic effect of temperatures of above 41°C, hyperthermia treatment in the temperature range of 39-43°C may also develop a cytotoxic effect on the congenital and adaptive immune system through indirect immunological effects.

For more than 30 years, attempts have been made to establish hyperthermia as a fixed and indisputable therapy procedure in multimodal tumour treatment. There are still insufficient clinical prospective studies with clearly defined issues and indication sectors, as well as adequate comparison groups to be compared and randomly selected with and without hyperthermia. In particular, also the target criteria of these studies must be carefully thought out, defined and observed with reference to patient-oriented use, also concerning the influence on long-term survival and on the quality of life.

As a preparation for a multi-centred Phase III study in private practices focusing on oncology and radiotherapy, the effectiveness of regional, deep hyperthermia in a respective matched-pair analysis will be compared in this work from the patient portfolio between 2005 and 2011 with reference to the effectiveness criteria (progression free survival and total survival). The cancer of the colon metastasised in the liver is chosen as a clinical picture. The fact that further organs are affected is not excluded, because, on the one hand, this can be taken into account in the matched-pair analysis and, on the other hand, in general with cancer of the colon the life time is only limited to a lesser extent in comparison with hepatic metastasis.

Regional, deep hyperthermia of the Oncotherm Company is used as the so-called Oncothermia without planning a magnetic resonance scanning or a control in the therapy. On the one hand, the reason for this is that these methods have been used since 2005 in the Bruch and Partners oncological Group practice in 3 locations in Bonn, Euskirchen and Rheinbach. On the other hand, the author is convinced that regional, deep hyperthermia can only be promoted as an additional pillar of tumour therapy if it is extensively and cost-efficiently available without the connection of a large device such as the magnetic resonance scanner.

1.1 Molecular and immunological effects of hyperthermia on tumour progression and metastasis

1.1.1 General activation of the immune system

The aim of deep hyperthermia is to achieve a temperature of 41-44°C over a period of at least 30 minutes, generally 60 minutes, in order to kill off tumour cells through the direct impact of heat.[1,2]

A further therapy principle of hyperthermia aims at getting a slight heating in the range of 39-40°C as the so-called fever therapy in order to achieve immunological effects. Whole-body hyperthermia treatments are mostly carried out within this fever-like temperature range, which in general are not as well tolerated as a regional deep hyperthermia.[3] Owing to this, whole-body hyperthermia is restricted to 1-2 applications, so that, in general, a long-term effect cannot be achieved.

Together with a stimulation of the adaptive immune response towards tumour-associated antigens, hyperthermia may boost the formation of

---

[1] Lepock, J.R.: *Role of nuclear protein denaturation and aggregation in thermal radiosensitization.* – Int J Hyperthermia 20(2004)115-130.

[2] Roti Roti, J.L.: *Cellular responses to hyperthermia (40-46 degrees C): Cell killing and molecular events.* – Int J Hyperthermia 24(2008)3-15.

[3] Skitzki, J.J., Repasky, E.A. and S.S. Evans: *Hyperthermia as an immunotherapy strategy for cancer.* – Curr Opin Invest Drugs 10(2009)550-558.

the so-called stress proteins (heat shock proteins) and further risk signals leading to the stimulation of congenital (innate) immune response.[4]

A release of immune-activating heat shock proteins in the extracellular milieu of tumour cells attracts antigen-presenting cells such as dendritic cells, monocytes and macrophages and stimulates their maturity. This causes the release of chemotactic active substances, which, in a further step, induce the migration of immune effector cells such as T lymphocytes to the tumour and their activation.

1.1.2 Temperature increase above 41 °C leading to death of tumour cells

With regional hyperthermia, only the tumour or a clinical relevant part of the tumour is subjected to heat treatment. It has been shown that cancer cells mainly kill off with temperatures in the range of 41-43°C. Normal tissue surrounding is not generally damaged by this.

The question then arises, why normal tissue proves to be more resistant towards increased temperatures compared with malign tissue.

Owing to their fast cell growth, it is necessary for tumours of more than 1mm^3 to build a new blood supply to the vessels (neo-angiogenesis). However, these tumour blood vessels are often defective in comparison to vessels in normal tissues and have a chaotic architecture.[5] Increased temperatures are normally regulated through an enhanced blood circulation in the tissue. Tumours with their irregular vessel architecture cannot transport warmth very well compared with normal tissues and therefore are exposed longer to the toxic effect of the heat.

---

[4] Lepock, J.R 2004, a.a.O.

[5] MOLLS, M., VAUPEL, P., NIEDER, C. AND M.S. ANSCHER: *The impact of tumour biology on cancer treatment and multidisciplinary strategies*. – In: BRADY, L.W., HEILMANN, H.P., MOLLS, M. AND J. J. NIEDER (eds.): *Medical radiology*. – Berlin, Heidelberg, New York, 2010, pp 117-128.

1.1.3 Synergy from hyperthermia and chemotherapy and/or radiotherapy

Regional hyperthermia is most effective if it is administered in combination with conventional forms of therapy such as chemotherapy and/or radiotherapy.

The "thermal enhancement ratio" from specific chemotherapy preparations reaches its maximum in a temperature range of 40.5- 43°C.[6] Targeted hyperthermia treatment is capable of transforming sub-lethal tumour cell damage of chemotherapy into death cells.[7]

In recent times, the effectiveness of thermosensitive liposomes in combination with hyperthermia has been tested in clinical protocols. Increased permeability of tumour vessels in combination with heat dependant release of chemotherapeutic agents from thermosensitive liposomes turn local hyperthermia into a therapeutic approach to guarantee targeted release of active ingredients on the tumour.[8]

Improved permeability of vessels also enables infiltration of the tumour with immune cells and may, in addition, enhance the efficiency of treatment based on anti-bodies[9] and nano particles.

---

[6] URANO, M., KURODA, M. AND Y. NISHIMURA: *For the clinical application of thermochemotherapy given at mild temperatures.* – Int J Hyperthermia 15(1999)79-107.

[7] MILLER, R.C., ROIZIN-TOWLE, L. AND K. KOMATSU: *Interaction of heat with x-rays and cis-platinum; cell lethality and oncogenic transformation.* – Int J Hyperthermia 5(1989)697-705.

[8] KONING, G.A., EGGERMONT, A.M. AND L.H. LINDNER: *Hyperthermia and thermosensitive liposomes for improved delivery of chemotherapeutic drugs to solid tumours.* – Pharm Res 27(2010)1750-1754.

[9] HOSONO, M., ENDO, K., UEDA, R. AND ONOYAMA, Y.: *Effect of hyperthermia on tumour uptake of radiolabeled anti-neural cell adhesion molecule antibody in small-cell lung cancer xenografts.* – J Nucl Med. 35(1994)504-9.

The highest extravasation of nano particles in tumour tissue is observed at a temperature of around 42°C.[10]

The synergistic effects of radiotherapy and hyperthermia are based especially on the improved blood flow achieved by the heat, and thus an enhanced supply of oxygen (oxygenisation) to the tumour.[11] Hypoxic tumour areas prove to be extremely resistant to radiation. Hyperthermia raises the permeability of vessels and thereby imparts an improved oxygen supply. Increased oxygen radicals may be formed in higher numbers in the tumour after radiation. These cause DNA damage in the tumour. Ideally, these finally lead to cell death.

1.1.4 Systemic effects of regional, deep hyperthermia

Molecular biological research works have proved in recent years that local therapy procedures such as local regional radiotherapy and regional deep hyperthermia may also develop systemic effects in terms of "abscopal effects".[12]

A possible mechanism of action of how local radiotherapy or thermal therapy may arouse systemic effects is the formation of forms of death of tumour cells. In turn, these could influence the immune system in different ways.

Figure 1 shows a schematic overview of how tumour cells that are killed off by means of chemotherapy, hyperthermia or radiotherapy contribute to inducing an anti-tumour response:

---

[10] KONG, G., BRAUN, R.D. AND M.W. DESWHRIST: *Characterization of the effect of hyperthermia on nanoparticle extravasation from tumour vasculature.* – Cancer Res 61(2001)3027-3032.

[11] OVERGAARD J.: *The current and potential role of hyperthermia in radiotherapy.* – Int J Rad Oncol Biol Phys 16(1989)535-549.

[12] DEMARIA, S., NG, B. AND M.L. DEVITT: *Ionizing radiation inhibition of distant untreated tumours (abscopal effect) is immune mediated.* – Int J Radiat Oncol Biol Phys 58(2004)862-870.

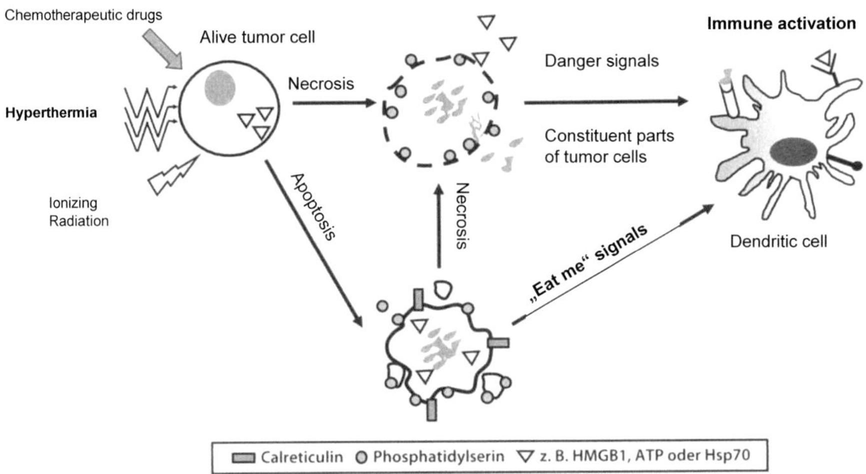

ATP: Adenosine-5′-triphosphate **HMGB1:** High-Mobility-Group Protein B1 **Hsp:** Heat Shock Protein

Figure 1: Immune activation by therapy-induced damaged tumour cells. Hyperthermia in combination with chemotherapy or radiotherapy induces tumour cell death[13]

The two main forms of cell death are apoptosis and necrosis. Cells at which the programmed cell death (apoptosis) have been induced, keep for many hours the integrity of their plasma membrane and go through characteristic changes in their protein and lipid composition in their cell surface.

The translocation and exposition of membrane phosphide phosphatidylserine from the inner to the outer cell membrane covering serves as an eat-me signal to macrophages, so eliminating apoptotic cells fast and effectively. The phagocytosis of apoptotic cells by macrophages leads to secretion of anti-inflammatory cytokines, which send only very weak signals to the immune system.[14]

[13] MULTHOFF, G. AND U. GAIPL: *Molekulare und immunologische Effekte der Hyperthermie auf Tumorprogression und Metastasierung.* – Der Onkologe 16(2010)1043-1051.

[14] VOLL, R.E., HERRMANN, M. AND E.A. ROTH: *Immunosuppressive effects of apoptotic cells.* – Nature 390(1997)350-351.

A secondary necrosis occurs if apoptotic cells of macrophages are not removed efficiently and if they lose the integrity of their plasma membrane in a second step and thus become necrotic.[15]

According to the Danger-hypothesis,[16] the immune system reacts in particular to signals released by the cells in necrosis. Water may infiltrate in necrotic cells by osmosis through tiny holes in the cell wall until the cell finally bursts. Uncontrolled release of intracellular localised proteins such as the high-mobility group box 1 protein (HMGB1), adenosine 5′-triphosphate or heat shock proteins occur by means of this process.

These extracellular components of necrotic tumour cells act as danger signals to the immune system: macrophages are attracted, they phagocyte the cell components and, contrary to the phagocytosis of apoptotic cells, release pro-inflammatory cytokines, which have a strong immunogenic effect on lymphocytes.[17]

Dendritic Cells (DC), cytotoxic T Lymphocytes (CTL) and natural killer cells (NK) are the central players of hyperthermia-induced immune-activation. Figure 2. Shows a scheme and a summary of the immune-activating effects of released Heat shock protein (Hsp 70) in the extracellular space by means of hyperthermia.

---

[15] SAVILL, J., DRANSFIELD, I. AND C. GREGORY: *Clearance of apoptotic cells regulates immune responses*. – Nat Rev Immunol 2(2002)965-975.
[16] MATZINGER, P.: *The danger model: A renewed sense of self*. – Science 296(2002)301-305.
[17] ANDREWS, N.W.: *Membrane repair and immunological danger*. – EMBO Rep. 6(2005)826-830.

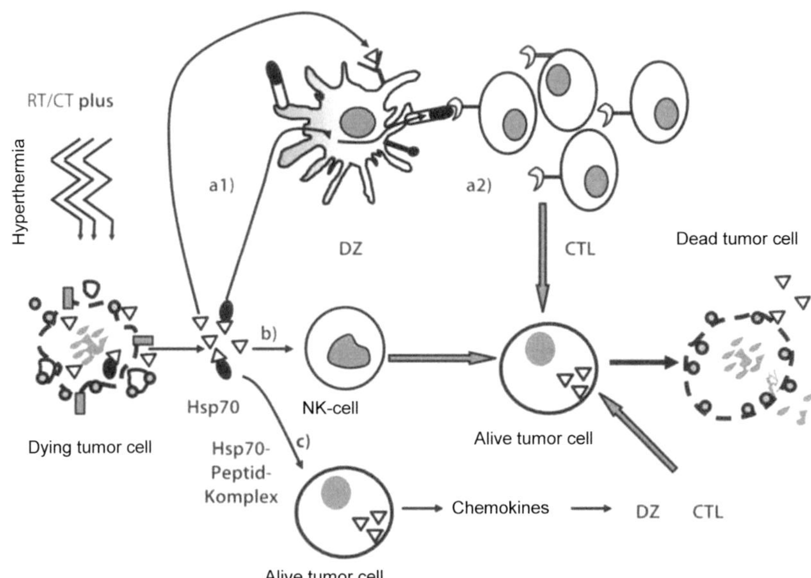

CT: Chemotherapy **DZ**: dendritic cell **Hsp**: Heat shock protein **NK-cell**: Natural killer cell **RT**: Radiotherapy

Figure 2[18]: Released Heat shock protein (Hsp 70) contributes to anti-tumour immunity. Combinations of chemotherapy and radiotherapy with hyperthermia lead to release of Hsp 70 and Hsp 70 peptide complexes

Hsp 70 produces a co-stimulation of DC, whereas the peptide complexes especially produce the absorption of tumour antigens and their cross-presentation through MHC-I molecules[19] (a1). The loaded DC then produces a specific activation and proliferation of CTL (a2). Hsp70 can also active NK cells direct, which attack tumour cells independent of MHC (b). Released Hsp70 and their peptide complexes may also have the effect of self-activation on tumour cells. Chemokines are released, which are responsible for attracting DC and CTL (c).

---

[18] MULTHOFF, G. AND U. GAIPL 2010, a.a.O.

[19] SHRIVASTAVA, P.K., CALLAHAN, M.K. AND M.M. MAURI: *Treating human cancers with heat shock protein-peptide complexes: The road ahead.* – Expert Opin Biol Ther 9(2009)179-186.

1.2 Physical and Technical Principles of Regional, Deep Hyperthermia

1.2.1 Definition of Terms[20]

A therapeutic rise in temperature from the normal body temperature to 40 up to 45 degrees Celsius is described as hyperthermia. Above 50 degrees Celsius, the term used is thermoablation.

The form of use and/or the area of treatment in which hyperthermia is used leads to a further classification:

Whole body hyperthermia (WBHT) heats the whole body, whereas this is heated at a range of temperatures of 39-40 degrees Celsius with a moderate whole body hyperthermia and with a range of temperatures from 41.8-42 degrees Celsius with extreme WBHT. Generally speaking, moderate WBHT is feasible without intensive medical care, whereas extreme WBHT is carried out under intensive supervision with narcotics or deep sedation.

Local regional hyperthermia (LRHT) heats only a defined tumour bearing area, either locally on the surface of the body up to a depth of 3 to 5cm or regionally, such as the pelvis or the area of the thigh. The so-called part-body hyperthermia (PBHT) represents a variety of this form of treatment, where the area warmed is a larger region, such as the whole abdomen. As a rule, the whole body temperature does not rise with these forms of treatment, or only slightly.

With interstitial hyperthermia (IHT), heat-generating applicators, such as radio-frequency antenna, are implanted, partly deep in the body. Small tumours are heated well with this kind of hyperthermia. Transferring this method to thermoablation is smooth, since, under protection

---

[20] Gellermann, J. and Wust, P.: *Physikalische und technische Grundlagen der regionalen Tiefenhyperthermie*. – Der Onkologe 16(2010)1052.

of the normal tissue, very high temperatures can be achieved in the vicinity of the applicators.

1.2.2 Thermal Dose[21]

As with radiotherapy, the thermal dose is defined in hyperthermia. In contrast to treatment with ionising radiation, where the pure physical dose in Gray (Gy) is used for determination of the dose, in hyperthermia, the equivalent time of the temperature reached at 43 degrees Celsius is used, the cumulative equivalent minutes at 43°C was (cem $_{43°C}$).[22] This corresponds rather to a biological dose than to a purely physical dose, because the temperature achieved is dependant not only on the radiant energy during hyperthermia, but also on the counter-regulation of the tissue treated. It is advantageous that with this information, especially with higher temperatures, a cytotoxic effect can be predicted to be good, similar to radiotherapy. The rule of thumb is that 60-90 mins at 43°C lead to an inactivation of 90% of the cells. The calculation can take place by means of the following form:

$$\text{cem}_{43°C} = t\,R^{(T-43)},$$

whereby t represents the time for a heating effect in minutes and T represents the temperature thereby reached. The factor, R, is 2 for all temperatures above 43°C and 4 for all temperatures below 43°C. This definition yields a doubling up of cem $_{43°C}$ for each rise by 1°C (above 43°C), in contrast to a quartering with each lowering by 1°C (below 43°C). 10 mins at 45°C correspond to a high thermal dose of 40 cem $_{43°C}$, by contrast 160 mins at 41°C correspond only to 10 cem $_{43°C}$.

---

[21] Ebd., 1053.

[22] SAPARETO, S.A. AND W.C. DEWEY: *Thermal dose determination in cancer therapy.* – Int J Radiat Oncol Biol Phys 10(1984)787-800.

1.2.3 Method of regional deep hyperthermia[23] in general and especially in oncothermia[24]

The regional deep hyperthermia method is based on the use of radio frequency waves. Indeed, it is possible for these to spread throughout the whole body, but they are differently transmitted through the different tissues and reflected or stopped at marginal surfaces between tissues of different electrical permeability, similar to light, which is differently transmitted through air and glass.

Therefore, regions with many different types of tissue tend to bundle the waves at some places, which may lead to overheating (the so-called "hot spots"), or to spread them, which may interfere with efficiency of the treatment ("cold spots").

Generally, bringing in radio waves can take place in different ways: by means of radiation through an antenna from the outside (radioactive), by means of a capacitive connection or by using magnetic alternating fields, which then secondarily generate an electrical field in the body.

As a rule, a cool water bolus is used for the optimised connection to the patient both with radioactive and with capacitive systems. The cool water bolus provides for an optimal transmission of energy, at the same time as taking the task of a superficial cooling system. The water is deionised in order for the radio wave not to be transferred into heat already in the bolus.

The frequency of the wave and thus its wave length in the body is a decisive aspect for the behaviour and the ability to focus of the radio waves. The higher the frequency of the radio wave is, the shorter is its wave length. In general, low wave lengths are used with a capacitive hyperthermia system, which accounts for the problem of focussing, by

---

[23] GELLERMANN, J. AND P. WUST 2010, a.a.O., 1054.

[24] SZASZ, A., SZASZ, N. AND O. SZASZ, O.: *Oncothermia: Principles and Practices.* – Berlin, Heidelberg, New York, 2011, pp. 174-242.

reason of the long wave lengths. The frequencies used in radioactive hyperthermia systems available in commerce are higher, but have a penetration depth of only 30cm, though good ability to focus.

The regional hyperthermia of Oncothermia is a capacitive-coupled energy transfer, forming the capacitor as the target. The capacitive-coupling technique is a relatively old technical solution.[25,26] In capacitive coupling, radiofrequency current flows through the patient from one electrode to the other (Figure 3).

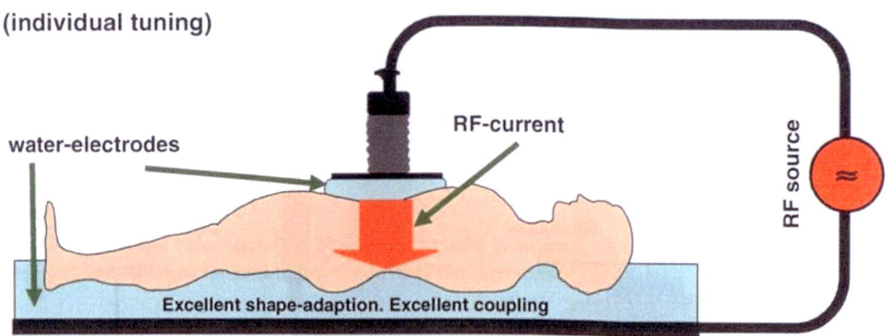

Figure 3: Patient is a part of the closed radiofrequency current circuit making oncothermia well controllable[27]

Electrodes are flat metals, both under a water pillow: one is in the bolus; one is under the water mattress. Water is a transmitter of the radiofrequency current, making a good fit of the human body to the flat metals possible. Both water electrodes (the water bed and the water bolus) are parts of the highly sophisticated electric circuit. The radiofrequency energy flows in a controlled way in the constrained directions. The current delivers the energy to the malignancy. Both electrodes are active, current flows through them in all the frequency periods.

---

[25] SONG, C.W., RHEE, J.G. AND C.K. LEE: *Capacitive heating of phantom and human tumors with an 8 MHz radiofrequency applicator (Thermotron RF-8).* – Int J Radiation Oncol Biol Phys 12(1986)365-372.

[26] HIRAOKA, M., JO, S. AND K. AKUTA: *Radiofrequency capacitive hyperthermia for deep-seated tumors* – I. Studies on thermometry. – Cancer 60(1987)121-127.

[27] SZASZ, A. et.al. 2011, a.a.O., p.175, Fig. 4.1.

The main advantage of Oncothermia is the large efficacy and less deep hot spots due to the pure electric field action. However, its disadvantage is unfortunately remarkable: surface (adipose) burn is more frequent than in the radioactive technical solution.

To choose the right frequency for Oncothermia the various components of the effects and practical applicability have to be considered. From these considerations the most important factors are:

- the request is to treat deeply reaching the body cross section, so the frequency for effective penetration depth must not to be higher than 25 MHz;
- to have an effect on the cellular membrane (i.e. at around 10 MHz);
- have the possibility of low frequency modulation (in a range up to 20 KHz), to use resonance effects (the carrier frequency must be at least 100-times higher than the modulation, for accurate info-transmitting, so the carrier frequency must be not less than 2 MHz);
- to be in a safe region, above the level for nervous excitations (more than 10 KHz) and below the level of microwave radiation (1 GHz).

Totalling all of the considerations above, it was practical for oncothermia to use a free frequency, which does not require shielding. The free frequencies are 13.56, 27.12 MHz, or 40.78 MHz in the requested regime. In comparison, at all of these there was a logical chance to choose the lowest possible for carrier frequency, namely 13.56 MHz.

This carrier frequency is fixed like the frequency of your favourite radio station, but it is only the basis, carrying the music and speech that you hear. The frequency 13.56 is only a carrier, which has information to transfer.

The fractal modulation (time fractal fluctuation) helps to select optimally between the malignant and healthy cells supported by the modulation-demodulation theory and experiments in humans though the modulation effect on living material is not free of scientific[28] and environmental political discussion related to "electrosmog pollution". The carrier frequency has three parameters fixing this radiation and can be modulated: its amplitude, frequency and phase (Figure 4).

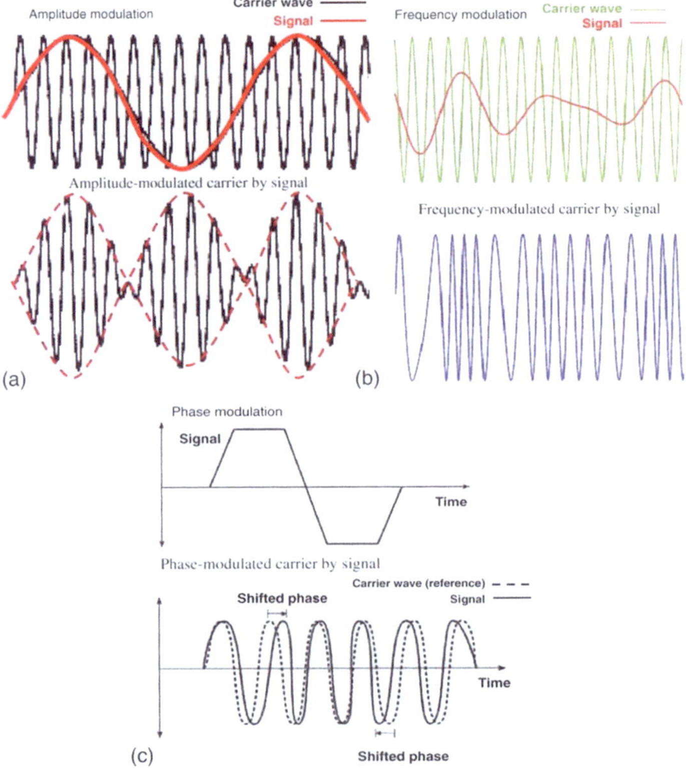

Figure 4: Modulations of Waves: Amplitude (AM), (a), frequency (FM), (b), and phase (PM), (c)[29]

The received modulated signal requires a demodulation (mining the info, detach the carrier). Definitely the easiest is the amplitude modulation-demodulation pair, because the modulation is only the change of

---

[28] *Proposed mechanism for the interaction of radiofrequency signals with living matter, demodulation in biological systems.* – Workshop, University of Rostock, Germany, 11-13 September 2006.

[29] SZASZ, A. et.al. 2011, a.a.O., p.175, Fig. 3.51.

the "strength" of the signal and the demodulation is a simple rectification, cutting the symmetric signal (Figure 5). All small amplitude modulations of the carrier frequencies (if the modulation is chosen on the stochastic resonance frequency) could cause a definite resonant effect on enzymatic processes and voltage ionic channels. Because of the very high number of such possible reactions in living organisms, these microscopic effects have a macroscopic result.

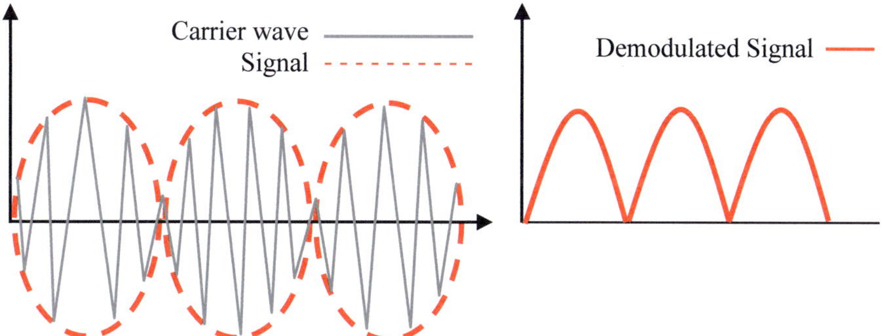

Figure 5: Demodulation of an amplitude-modulated signal. The process involves "cutting" the negative part (rectification)

The 13.56-MHz RF frequency carries energy to heat, but its effect is indefinite in its target. It heats up everything along the path of the conduction, and the heat flows into the neighbourhood by heat diffusion and active blood flow, seeking to equalise the temperature all over the body. These conditions request additional and effective selection factors to the above-described impedance selection, for example by modulation. The modulated carrier frequency performs a selective energy delivery to make the cell killing optimal in a mostly apoptotic way.

A special modulation[30] based on a pink-noise power spectrum is applied in the oncothermia process to enhance the collective apoptotic control of cell death.[31]

---

[30] SZASZ, A. et.al. 2011, a.a.O., p. 468, Appendix 29.

[31] SZENDRO, P., VINCZE, G. AND A. SZASZ: *Bio-Response on white-noise-excitation.* – Electromagn Biol Med 20(2001)215-229.

Hyperthermia generates high-amplitude voltage-peaks to make the dielectrophoretic (cataphoric) effects and all the voltage-dependent factors effective. The pink noise is the self-organising fluctuation, the operating noise of homeostasis. The essence of this is the random physiological effects that are collectively controlled by their spectrum deviation which is constant in homeostasis. This externally constrained fluctuation promotes the collectivity, constrains to equalise the deviations of the random events. The collectivity is expressed by the cellular communications in living organisms (adherence, junctions) controlled by this modulation method. The deviation control is the original pink noise having a zero-frequency centre, so the demodulation of the modulated signal is essential (stochastic resonance mechanism, window of action).

The oncothermia system has a reaction-promoting behaviour as catalysts do. To damage and destroy the membrane a temperature over 42°C is required to exceed the energy barrier of the membrane stability. In oncothermia this barrier is suppressed, a lower temperature (lower thermal energy) is then required to carry out the requested action (Fig. 6).

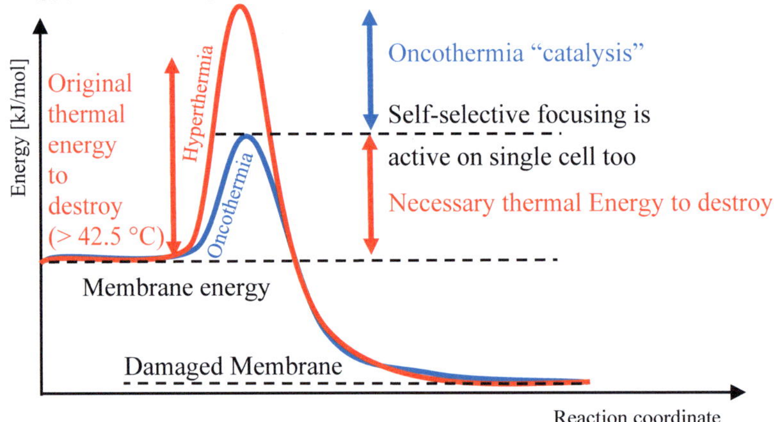

Figure 6: Modulation helps to suppress the energy barrier needed for membrane damage[32]

---

[32] SZASZ, A. et.al. 2011, a.a.O., p.222, Fig. 4.53. (Nachbildung)

This different efficacy of hyperthermia and oncothermia is demonstrated in experimental cell models (HepG2 cell line: dynamic development of ß-catenin as indicator of apoptosis with time after treatment) (Fig. 7) and xenograft models (Fig 8). Even at a lower temperature of 38°C oncothermia is more as hyperthermia at 42°C in experimental models (Fig. 9).

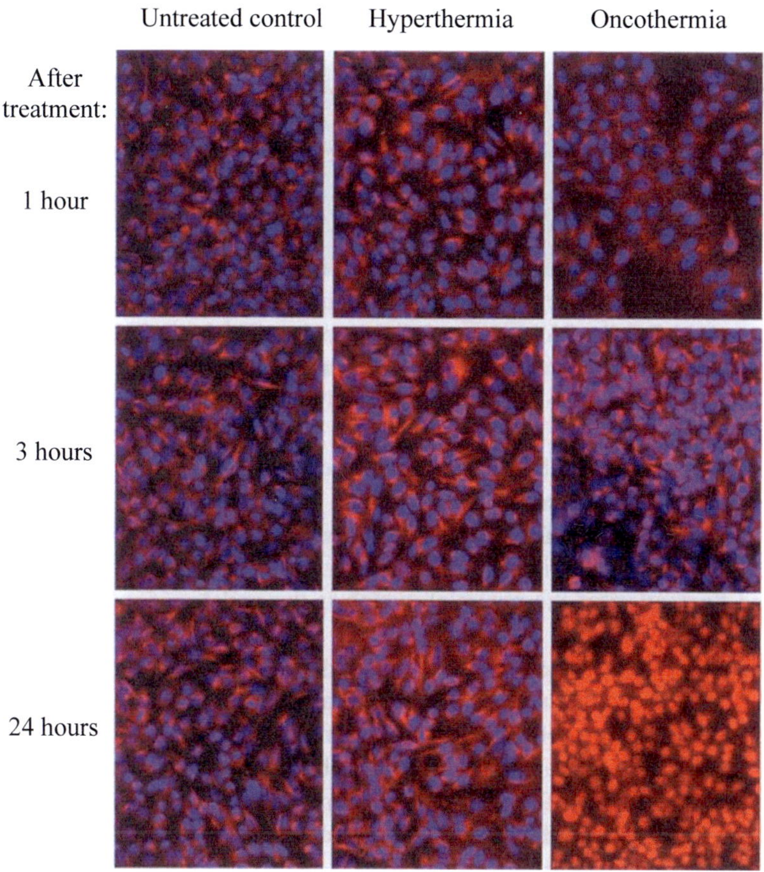

Figure 7: Development of ß-catenin with time elapsed after treatment in untreated, hyperthermia and oncothermia-treated samples. (Immuno-fluorescent microscopic images, red: ß-catenin, blue: cell nuclei)[33]

---

[33] ANCOCS, G., SZASZ, O. AND A. SZASZ: *Oncothermia treatment of cancer: for the laboratory to clinic*. – Electromagn Biol Med 28(2009)148-165.

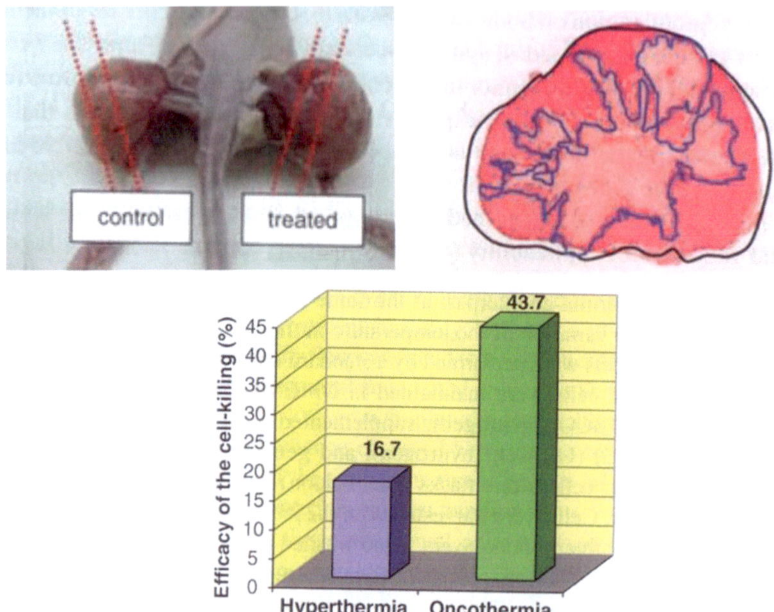

Figure 8: Macroevaluation of the efficacy of oncothermia in comparison with hyperthermia in HT29 tumour xenograft in nude mouse. Change of the areas of dead and vivid parts as a percentage of the untreated control for the same experimental animal (data average of three animals each)[34]

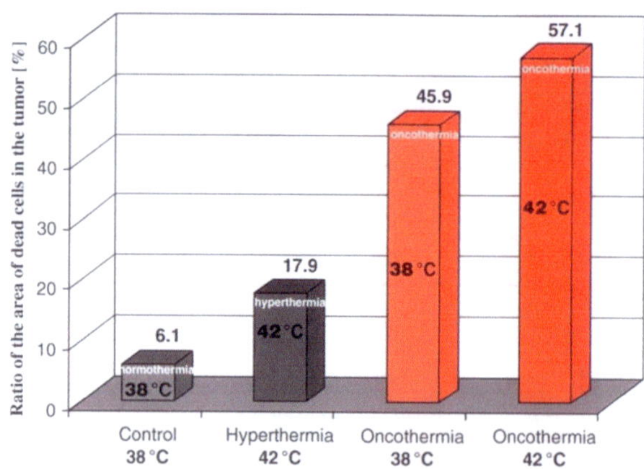

Figure 9: Ratio of the dead cells in the studied tumours, evaluated by morphological methods[35]

[34] SZASZ, A. et.al. 2011, a.a.O., p.228, Fig. 4.59.

[35] SZASZ, A. et.al. 2011, a.a.O., p.238, Fig. 4.76.

A comparison of hyperthermia and oncothermia combined both methods with Mitomycin-C (MMC) single-dose chemotherapy in vivo at tissue and cellular level: HT 29 human colo-rectal carcinoma cell line-derived xenograft tumour model in nude mouse: for hyperthermia (42 C) +3mg/kg MMC i.p. (30 min before the treatment) and for oncothermia (42 C) + 3mg/kg MMC i.p. (30 min before the treatment). The relative difference (both compared to its control average) is shown in Fig 10.

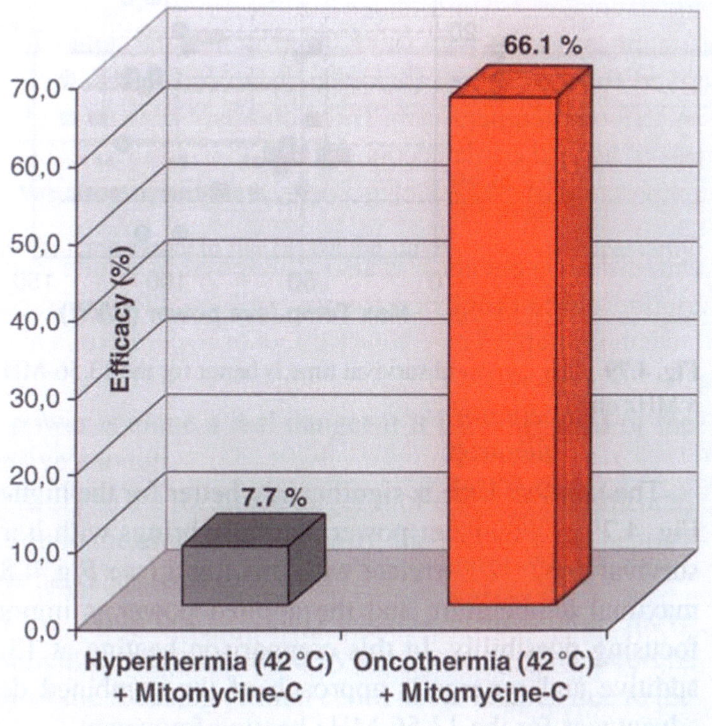

Figure 10: Experimental comparison of hyperthermia with Mitomycin-C and oncothermia with the same dose Mitomycin-C, cell killing is relative to the control tumour in the same animal (the values are from 2 animals/4 tumours)[36]

---

[36] SZASZ, A. et.al. 2011, a.a.O., p.239, Fig. 4.78.

1.3 The significance of regional deep hyperthermia within drug tumour therapy

Based on existing evidence from in vitro examinations, it arises that hyperthermia indeed has a per se cytotoxic effect above a threshold temperature (breakpoint temperature) of 42.5 Celsius degrees owing to the temperature increase, and the cytotoxic effect follows the dose-effect principle (Arrhenius analysis based on multi-target single-hit model for the mathematical description of heat survival curves after a single hyperthermia exposure).[37] Until the end of the 1990s, the thermal iso-effect dose concept (TID) was valid, from which the equivalent doses were derived for the clinical treatment in accordance with the killing rates with different temperatures.[38] The dogma was that the clinical effectiveness of hyperthermia is connected with a homogeneous distribution of temperature of ≥42.5 Celsius degrees in the tumour.

To this end, the TID concept was also transferred by single analogy for the description of the efficiency analysis of hyperthermia in combination with chemotherapy. The primary effect of hyperthermia as thermosensitisation for cytostatic effective substances was classified below this breakpoint temperature of 42.5 degree Celsius. Taking into account the complexity of pleiotropic interactions below this breakpoint temperature of 42.5 degree Celsius, between hyperthermia and chemotherapy, as an in vivo therapy concept, led to revision of the method of approach and to a new orientation in clinical studies, because the effect of milieu factors, the perfusion changes and the cellular sensitisation to cytostatic drugs had not been determined hitherto, at the place of the overheating in the quantitative description of index temperatures, or thermal dose equivalents.

---

[37] Bauer, K.D. and K.J. Henle: *Arrhenius analysis of heat survival curves form normal and thermotolerant CHO cells*. – Radiat Res 78(1979)251-263.

[38] Dewey, W.C.: *Arrhenius relationships from the molecule and cell to clinic*. – Int J Hyperthermia 10(2009)457-483.

According to the concept at the time, the temperature-dependant enhancement of the cytotoxic effect of chemotherapy thus has two essential components:

- a direct, temperature-dependant cytotoxic effect at ≥42.5 degree Celsius and
- an interaction with the anti-tumour effective substance on target structures in the tumour cell (40-43 degree Celsius).

It can also be understood with this that at diverse distribution of temperatures in the tissue of the tumour, both components are added in separate areas and are responsible for the total effect of hyperthermia.

The mechanisms for improving the effectiveness of cytostatic drugs in their interactions with hyperthermia are varied.[39] With the help of isobologram analysis, the dose-effect examinations in cell cultures or in animal models enable the phenomenological description of the type of interaction (independent, additive or synergistic) with hyperthermia for various cytostatic drugs. A striking aspect is that, for the most part, only low increasing effectiveness is observed under hypothermal conditions for anti-metabolic, cytostatic effective drugs (such as Fluorouracil 5FU and Methotrexate). Also, the so-called Taxane group of drugs (Paclitaxel and Docetaxel) show no intensifying effects (independent effect). An additive effect occurs with the raising of the temperature for alkylating substances (such as Cyclophosphamide and Ifosfamide) and for nitrosourea compounds as well as for anthracyclines. This effect is limited only to a closely circumscribed range of 40-41 degrees Celsius (threshold effect) for Doxorubicin. It is important for some cytostatic drugs that the enhancing effect takes place depending on the sequence

---

[39] DAHL, O.: *Interaction of hyperthermia and chemotherapy.* – Recent Results Cancer Res 107(1988)157-169.

of the application[40], which has already been also taken into account in clinical studies (hyperthermia 24 hours after administration of Gemzar).

An exponential increase in the total effectiveness (synergistic effect) can be proved for other cytostatic drugs (i.e. platin derivatives).

By reason of early results from radio-biological basic research, which made clear an increase in the radiotherapeutic effects on cells and tissue (inhibiting DNA repair systems, especially thermo-sensitisation of hypoxic cells and S phase cells, re-oxygenation of tumour tissue by increased perfusion) by raising the temperature, clinical Phase II/III studies had been carried out since the mid-1980s, in combination with hyperthermia and radiotherapy.[41] A recently published Cochrane Review has analysed available data on treatment of locally advanced rectal carcinoma with reference to simultaneous hyperthermia and radiotherapy.[42] A current study is also recruting volunteers with reference to the issue of radiotherapy with accompanying hyperthermia for locally advanced rectal carcinoma (PI Dr. Oliver Ott, Erlangen, EurdraCT 2009-010093-38).

Interest in oncology about drug therapy for tumours, in combination with hyperthermia, is based on the enhancing effect shown, by means of hyperthermia on many cytostatic effecting cancer medicines, which are used clinically in standard treatment protocols. In addition, the observation that also primary chemo-resistant cells unanimously show a high thermo-sensitisation, and that an induced chemo resistance can be

---

[40] HAVEMAN, J., RIETBROEK, R.C. AND A. GEERDINK: *Effect of hyperthermia on the cytotoxicity of 2′,2′-difluorodeoxycytidine (gemcitabine) in cultured SW1573cells.* – Int J Cancer 62(1995)627-630.

[41] OTT, J.O., SCHMIDT, M., AND R. SAUER: *Bedeutung der Hyperthermie im Rahmen radioonkologischer Behandlungsstrategien.* – Der Onkologe 16(2010)1072-1078.

[42] DE HAAS-KOCK, D.F., BUIJSEN, J. AND M. PIJLS-JOHANNESMA: *Concomitant hyperthermia and radiation therapy for treating locally advanced rectal cancer.* – Cochrane Database Syst Rev CD006269, 2009.

overcome under hyperthermal conditions for the same cytostatic drug, was of pioneering importance.[43]

As a result of this knowledge, prospective studies on systemic or regional chemotherapy in combination with various hyperthermia procedures were also carried out in the mid-1990s.

The technical further developments in the area of regional deep hyperthermia (oncothermia: Hungary, RF-8-Thermotron: Japan, BSD-System: USA), the initial description of the HIPEC procedure (Sugarbaker, USA), the intracavitary microwave procedures (Synergo 101-1: Netherlands) and the hyperthermal isolated organ perfusion (HIP) procedure allowed in addition increasing recruiting of patients with deep-seated tumours in the abdominal and groin areas in these studies.

Published Phase II and III studies on hyperthermia in combination with chemotherapy normally carried out intensively on pre-treated patients with solid tumours are listed in Tables 1 and 2 below.

TABLE 1: PHASE II STUDIES ON HYPERTHERMIA COMBINED WITH CHEMOTHERAPY

Authors	Tumour	Patient Number	Treatment	Results (Response)
Romanowski 1993[44]	Paediatric sarcoma	34	VP 16 + IFO + Carbo	7 CR ("best response"), Duration 7-64 months

[43] TOWLE, L.R.: *Hyperthermia and drug resistance*. – In: URANO, M. AND E. DOUBLE (eds.): *Hyperthermia and oncology*. Vol. 4. – Utrecht, 1989, pp. 91-113.

[44] ROMANOWSKI, R., SCHÖTT, C. AND R. ISSELS, R.: *Regionale Hyperthermie mit systemischer Chemotherapie bei Kindern und Jugendlichen: Durchführbarkeit und klinische Verläufe bei 34 intensiv vorbehandelten Patienten mit prognostisch ungünstigen Tumorerkrankungen*. –Klin Padiatr 205(1993)249-256..

Wessalowski 2003[45]	Paediatric germ cell tumours and sarcoma	39	CDDP + VP 16 + IFO (PEI)	20 CR + 10 PR (77%)
Rietbroek 1997[46]	Cervix cancer	23	CDDP weekly	2 pCR/1 CR + 9 PR (52 %)
Franckena 2007[47]	Cervix cancer	47	CDDP weekly	3 CR + 23 PR (58%)
Jones 2005[48]	Ovarian cancer FIGO III/IV, platinum-resistant 90%	41	CDDP intraperitoneal HT	10 CR + 8 PR (44%), OS: 33 months
Fotopoulou 2010[49]	Ovarian cancer FIGO III/IV, platinum-resistant 80%	36	Liposomal doxorubicin (Caelyx) or carboplatin or Topotecan combined with RHT	1 CR + 12 PR (36%), OS: 12 months
Atmaca 2009[50]	Relapsed ovarian cancer	47	Carbo combined with WBH	PR 45%

45 WESSALOWSKI, R., SCHNEIDER, D.T. AND O. MILS: *An approach for cure: PEI-chemotherapy and regional deep hyperthermia in children and adolescents with unresectable malignant tumors*. – Klin Padiatr 215(2003)303-309.

46 RIETBROEK, R.C., SCHILTHUIS, M.S. AND P.J.M. BAKKER: *Phase II trial of weekly locoregional hyperthermia and cisplatin in patients with a previously irradiated recurrent carcinoma of the uterine cervix*. – Cancer 79(1997)935-943.

47 FRANCKENA, M., STALPERS, L.J. AND P.C. KOPER, P.C.: *Long-term improvement in treatment outcome after radiotherapy and hyperthermia in locoregionally advanced cervix cancer: an update of the Dutch Deep Hyperthermia Trial*. – Int J Radiat Oncol Biol Phys 70(2008)1176-1182.

48 JONES, E., SECORD, A.A. AND L.R. PROSNITZ: *Intraperitoneal cisplatin and whole adbomen hyperthermia for relapsed ovarian carcinoma*. – Int J Hyperthermia 22(2006)161-172.

49 FOTOPOULOU, C., CHO, C.H. AND R. KRAETSCHELL: *Regional abdominal hyperthermia combined with systemic chemotherapy for the treatment of patients with ovarian cancer relapse: results of a pilot study*. – Int J Hyperthermia 26(2010)118-126.

50 ATMACA, A., AL BATRAN, S.E., AND A. NEUMANN: *Whole-body hyperthermia in combination with carboplatin in patients with recurrent ovarian cancer – a Phase II study*. – Gynaecol Cancer 112(2009)384-388.

Gofrit 2004[51]	Superficial bladder cancer Ta-T1 G3	24	MMC and intravesical HT	LPFS: 62,5%, follow-up 35 months
Witjes 2009[52]	Superficial bladder cancer G3 (CIS)	51, 34 BCG-refractory	MMC and intravesical HT	CR: 92%, LPFS: 50% Follow up 27 Months
Authors	Tumour	Patient Number	Treatment	Results (Response)

Abbreviations: WBH whole body hyperthermia, RHT regional hyperthermia, HT hyperthermia, CR complete remission, PR partial remission, DFS disease free survival, LPFS local progression free survival, OS overall survival, VP 16 Etoposide, IFO Ifosfamide, Carbo Carboplatin, CDDP Cisplatin, MMC Mitomycin C.

TABLE 2: PHASE III STUDIES ON HYPERTHERMIA COMBINED WITH CHEMOTHERAPY

Authors	**Tumour**	**Patient Number**	**Treatment**	**Results (Response)**
Colombo 2003[53]	Superficial bladder carcinoma Ta-T1 G3	83	MMC + intravesical HT vs. MMC	LPFS 57,5 vs. 17,1%, p=0,0002
Issels 2010[54]	High-risk soft tissue sarcoma	341	Preoperative EIA, Op, Radiatio, postoperative EIA, randomized +/- HT	DFS p=0,011, HR 0,70; OS p=n.s., OS n=269 per protocol n=0,038 HR, 066

Abbreviations: RHT regional hyperthermia, CR complete remission, PR partial remission, DFS disease free survival, LPFS local progression free survival, OS overall survival, MMC Mitomycin C, E Etoposid, I Ifosfamid, A Doxorubicin

---

[51] GOFRIT, O.N., SHAPIRO, A. AND D. PODE: *Combined local bladder hyperthermia and intravesical chemotherapy for the treatment of high-grade superficial bladder cancer.* –Urology 63(2004)466-471.

[52] WITJED, J.A., HENDRICKSEN, K. AND O. GOFRIT: *Intravesical hyperthermia and mitomycin-C for carcinoma in situ of the urinary bladder: experience of the European Synergo® working party.* – World J Urol 27(2009)319-324.

[53] COLOMBO, R., DA POZZO, L.F. AND A. SALONIA: *Multicentric study comparing intravesical chemotherapy alone and with local microwave hyperthermia for prophylaxis of recurrence of superficial transitional cell carcinoma.* – J Clin Oncol 21(2003)4270-4276.

[54] ISSELS, R.D., LINDNER, L.H. AND J. VERWEIJ: *Neo-adjuvant chemotherapy alone or with regional hyperthermia for locolised high-risk soft-tissue sarcoma: a randomised Phase 3 multicentre study.* – Lancet Oncol 11(2010)561-570.

The review of these completed Phase II/III studies of hyperthermia combined with chemotherapy shows, on the one hand, "proof of efficacy" of the special clinical problem and, on the other hand, "proof of concept" for further therapy studies and, therefore, it has also motivated the author to carry out this pilot study on a new question of this multimodal therapy, involving chemotherapy and hyperthermia, also in the author's patients, because studies on the question whether a survival advantage is obtained with the addition of hyperthermia to standard chemotherapy with liver metastases originated in the colorectal area, have not been published.

Concerning the question of adding chemotherapy to the non-standard treatment of mono hyperthermia in the case of liver metastases originated in the colorectal area in the refractory (n=80)[55] situation, a small German study did not show any significant survival advantage between the groups. However, a trend to a clear survival advantage was shown in an historic comparison (Fig. 11).

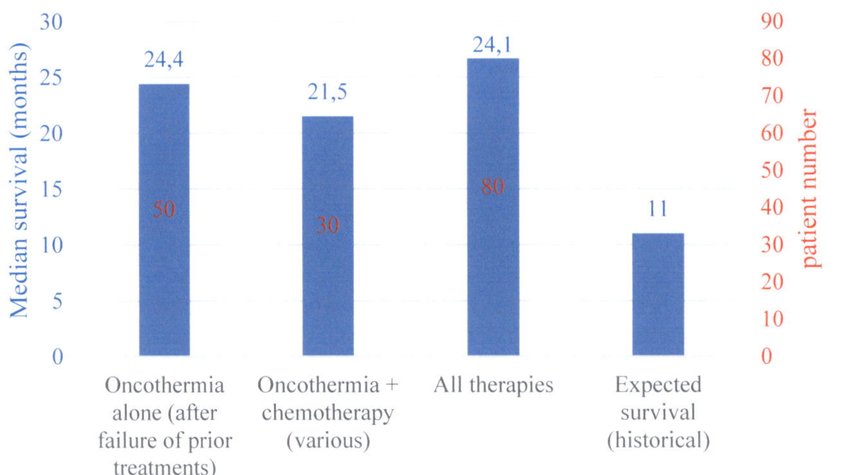

Figure 11: Median survival for patients having combined chemotherapy with oncothermia or monotherapy with oncothermia[55]

---

[55] HAGER, E.D.: *Deep hyperthermia with radiofrequencies in patients with liver metastases from colorectal cancer.* – Anticancer Res 19(1999)3404-3408. (Neugestaltung)

This study may be criticised for no chemotherapy substance with significant effect enhanced by hyperthermia being used on a large number of patients (65% 5-FU and Leucovorin).

In a further small German pilot study, so far published only in abstract form, which went into the question of the effectiveness of chemotherapy in the 1st line and/or chemotherapy and hyperthermia (oncothermia) in the 2nd line (n=15), in the case of the use of new substances (Oxaliplatin and Irinotecan) with the property of effect enhancing by means of hyperthermia, an improvement in local response rates of 51% (Oxaliplatin and 5 FU/folinic acid) to 80% (Irinotecan and Capecitabine) (Fig 12) was shown, without significantly increased additional toxicity in the second line arm, with additional hyperthermia.[56]

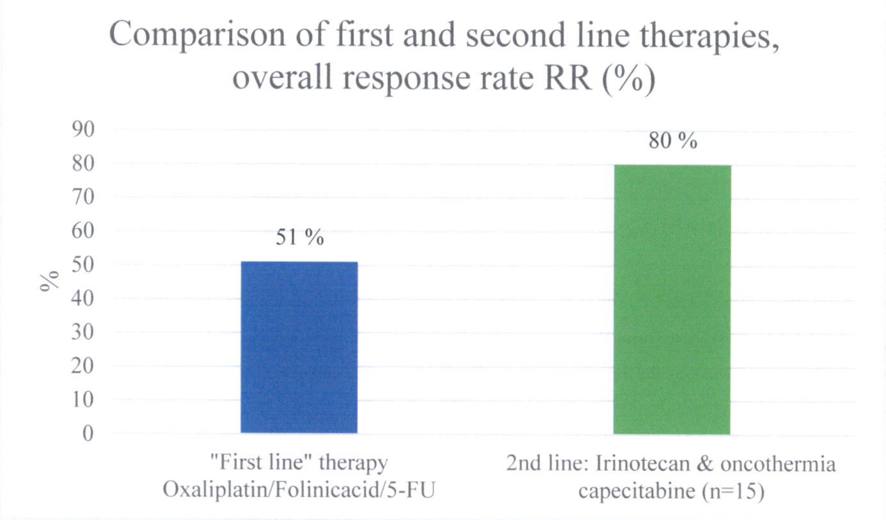

Figure 12: Local response rate was higher in second line treatment with complementary oncothermia application[56]

[56] PANAGIOTOU, P., SOSADA, M., SCHERING, S. AND H. KIRCHNER: *Irinotecan plus capecitabine with regional electrohyperthermia of the liver as second line therapy in patients with metastatic colorectal cancer.* – ESHO, Jun 8-11. 2005, Graz, Austria. (Nachbildung)

2. Matched-pair analysis of patients with hepatic metastatic carcinoma of the colon (chemotherapy on the liver with and without regional deep hyperthermia)

2.1 Problem

It was possible for the survival rates of patients with colorectal carcinoma and liver metastases (palliative situation) to be increased by means of adding new substances and antibodies to 5FU based chemotherapy within the drug therapy of tumours from 6 months to 20-24 months on average, and it indicates certain plateau building in the improvement of palliative therapy options.

Apart from this, the trend towards multi-modal treatment in oncology is recognised, which combines procedures of drug treatment for tumours with those without drugs, to achieve better survival rates for patients. Examples of these are the addition of radiotherapy in adjuvant and neoadjuvant treatment situations and the local ablative procedures within liver metastases operations or liver metastasis ablation by means of radiation (body stereotaxy), thermo or cryo ablation.

Local regional deep hyperthermia has shown promising results in preclinical and first clinical studies, also with the examined subject of colorectal carcinoma, as mentioned above. Therefore, it appears justified to the author to test out in a pilot study, whether adding local regional hyperthermia for the treatment of liver metastasis of patients with colorectal carcinoma leads to an improvement in survival under standard medication treatment.

A Phase III Study with identical chemotherapy, including the new drugs and identical antibody treatment (Bevacizumab and Cetuximab), indeed appeared to the author to be an ideal test environment, because, as mentioned above, there exist a Phase II study with historic comparison group and a Phase II study with comparison of the use of hyperthermia in second-line treatment. This indeed appeared to the author to be basically possible by reason of the necessary number of patients and in view of the inflow into 3 oncology focused practices (Bonn, Euskirchen, Rheinbach) treating patients from 5 hospitals without oncology departments (Marienhospital in Euskirchen, Malteser-Krankenhaus in Bonn/Rhein-Sieg, St.-Marien-Hospital in Bonn, St.-Josef-Hospital in Bonn-Beuel, Dreifaltigkeitskrankenhaus in Wesseling). But an argument against that was the steady further development of chemo-immunotherapy and the basic impossibility in the palliative situation to be able to give identical drug therapy to all study patients, having an existing portfolio of patients of elderly biological age levels and comorbidities of an oncological group. Also the difficulty in defining a drug combination as a standard treatment in the palliative situation, and the development of drug therapy within the period of the study, were two arguments against such a Phase III study.

The author has so far opted for a comparison of the respective therapy, best possibly used according to the existing biological function of the patient in combination with the local regional electro-hyperthermia of the liver. The author also compares this group with a matched-pair group, each having received an identical chemo-immunotherapy (containing 5-FU or Capecitabine and possibly any new substance plus antibodies, if necessary) at the time of forming the pairs. In order for the bias factors to be minimised, when possible, Irinotecan was used as a modern substance, and Bevacizumab as an antibody.

An improvement of the progression-free survival (PFS) was the primary target criterion. Indeed, the entire survival was recorded, but an improvement of the same was only a secondary target owing to the diverse recurrent treatments available.

2.2 Group of patients (original data, see Appendix)

During the period of 1/1/2005 to 30/6/2011, 50 patients with hepatic, metastatic colorectal carcinoma were treated only with systemic cytostatic therapy (chemotherapy, if necessary combined with antibody therapy), in first therapy line, because of liver metastasis (25 patients), Group A, and with chemotherapy in first therapy line, because of liver metastasis and additional local regional hyperthermia of the liver (25 patients), Group B. Under this therapy, the treatment was carried out up to progression.

The selection of the treatment took place by chance after advising all patients on the option of supplementing chemotherapy with hyperthermia, irrespective of their insurance status and irrespective of whether there was an acceptance of the costs by the insurance company. When there was no acceptance of the costs by the insurance company, the costs of treatment were borne by the practice, in order to exclude social bias, as far as possible.

A retrospective matched-pair analysis with formation of pairs with reference to the diagnosis (carcinoma of the colon or carcinoma of the rectum), the stage of the tumour and the chemo-antibody therapy used, took place. The addition of the initial stage of the tumour took place for taking into account the biology of the tumour (grading and growth of the tumour at the time of the first diagnosis).

No allocation of pairs was made with reference to pre-treatment with a first diagnosis, to gender and age, as well as to existing accompanying diseases.

2.3 Hyperthermia

A local regional electro-hyperthermia of the liver was carried out with the 30cm probe of the EHY-2000plus, oncothermia device of the Oncotherm company, twice weekly (once on the day of chemotherapy, once 48 hours later), each for 60 minutes. 60-140 Watts were applied with Rife (frequency modulation). Technical data: System voltage: AC 230V/50Hz/Driving power: 1600 VA/Maximum power output: max. 150 W/Nominal load: 50 Ohms/output carrier frequency: 13.56 (MHz)/Modulated output frequency: fractal noise.

2.4 Chemotherapy

Chemotherapy was not homogeneous. All combinations used normally in palliative chemotherapy on colorectal carcinoma were possible. Selection took place in accordance with the volume of the tumour, comorbidity and side-effects profile. As a rule, a chemo-continuous infusion containing 5-FU (2600mg/m2 for 24 hours modulated by means of folinic acid in accordance with the Working Association of Internal Medicine/Oncology (AIO)) or Capecitabine (1250mg/m2 twice daily for 14 days followed by a break of 7 days) plus a new substance (Irinotecan, Oxaliplatin, with intolerance, Mitomycin) plus, if there was no contraindication, the VEGF antibody, Bevacizumab, for 6 weeks, followed by a break of 2 weeks.

2.5 Results

All in all, 50 patients with liver metastases and colorectal carcinoma were treated systemically with chemotherapy and/or chemo-antibody therapy in the first-line. 25 (group A) were treated with hyperthermia and 25 (group B) without.

Liver metastasis appeared in an average of 173 (group A) against 177 weeks (group B) after the first diagnosis of colorectal carcinoma, whereas the liver metastasis already appeared synchronically with the first diagnosis of 60 against 56%.

Pre-treatment consisted of a continuous infusion (if necessary with radiotherapy within the Erlanger protocol of each 2/25) containing FU for 8/25 (group A) and 9/25 (group B) in the course of the first diagnosis and/or a combination of FU and Oxaliplatin (generally adjuvant to the FOLFOX4 protocol[57]).

---

[57] De Gramont, A., Figer, A. and Seymour, M.: *Leucovorin and fluorouracil with or without oxaliplatin as first-line treatment in advanced colorectal cancer.* – J Clin Oncol 18(2000)2938-47.

There was no additional organ metastasis (lungs, other abdominal organs) of large significance (>5cm tumour mass) (each group 2/25=8%) and no significant difference in extent between pairs.

On average, the patients in the group with systemic therapy were 65 (39-74 range) and 71 (52-86) in the group with additional hyperthermia.

20% of the women (5/25) were treated with a combined therapy and 40% of the women (10/25) were treated only with chemotherapy. This difference is explained by the insurance status of the women, who are generally insured through the statutory insurance system and were willing to accept sponsoring by the practice only to a limited extent.

In comparison, the men often received above-average governmental health support, because of their civil servant status in the city of Bonn and surroundings, or were privately insured. Consequently these institutions generally bear the costs of hyperthermia.

Chemotherapy was exclusively based on 5 FU in both groups by 5/25 (28%) patients, whereas 18/25 (72%) received a modern substance (28% Oxaliplatin, 40% Irinotecan, 4% Mitomycin).

Bevacizumab was used as antibody in addition to chemotherapy in both groups, 15/25 (60%). Cetuximab was not used, because there was no first-line approval at the start of the study.

Hyperthermia was applied with the large probe at an average of 140 Watts over an average of 17 sessions (range of 2-54).

As a main target criterion, progression-free survival (PFS) was on average 66.6 weeks with hyperthermia and 41.8 weeks without. Total survival was on average 104.0 weeks with hyperthermia, and 60.4 weeks without. It was now necessary to clarify whether this advantage of 37 or 40% achieved statistical significance.

The data of Mr. Benjamin Mayer, Institute of Epidemiology and Medical Biometry, University of Ulm, Schwabstr. 13, 89075 Ulm, Director Prof. Dr. Rainer Muche, were presented in order to analyse the study configuration (case control study with matching tumour (colon or rectum); tumour stage, type of chemo-immunotherapy).

The first analysis of progression-free survival (PFS), analysis on 2/11/2011 (Benjamin Mayer, Institute of Epidemiology and Medical Biometry, University of Ulm, Schwabstr. 13, 89075 Ulm, Director: Prof. Dr. Rainer Muche) resulted in the following Kaplan-Meier curve:

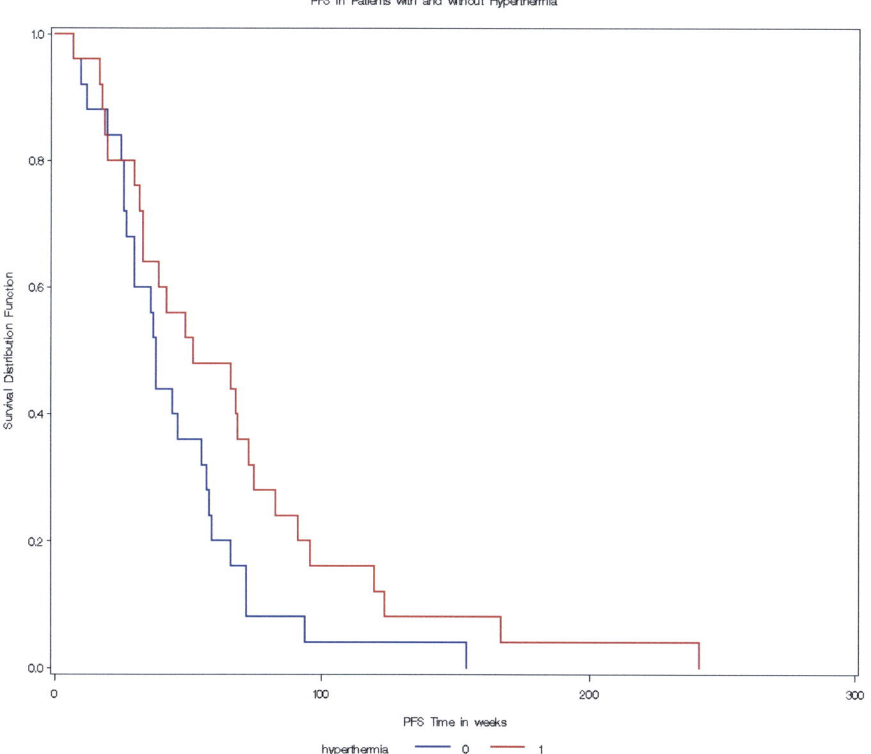

Log-rank test result:
p-value = 0.0633

Result of Cox model for the calculation of HR:
HR = 0.582
95% confidence interval: [0.326,1.042]
p-value = 0.0683

Analysis of overall survival , abbreviated as OS, Analysis on 2/11/2011 (Benjamin Mayer, Institute of Epidemiology and Medical Biometry, University of Ulm, Schwabstr. 13, 89075 Ulm, Director: Prof. Dr. Rainer Muche):

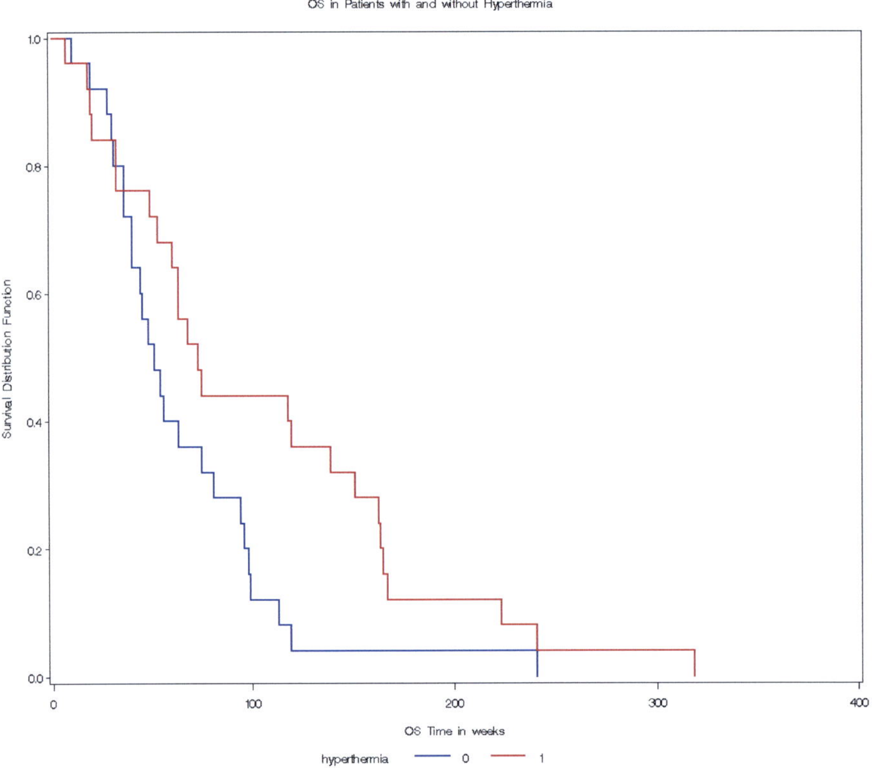

Log-rank test result:
p-value = 0.0341

Result of Cox model for the calculation of HR:
HR = 0.539
95% confidence interval: [0.299,1.971]
p-value = 0.0397

A strong tendency that patients profited from local regional hyperthermia, both for PFS and for OS, was shown in the assessment of statistics of the first analysis.

The log-rank test results were not supposed to be overestimated in both cases because the corresponding survival time functions overlap and therefore, there are no optimal conditions for the use of the log-rank test. However, the p-values of the log-rank test in both cases are confirmed by the results of the Cox model. It was suggested to use the Cox model p-values for the work.

The HRs show both for PFS and for OS that patients without local regional hyperthermia have an almost doubly high risk of an event (progression and/or death). In other words: patients with local regional hyperthermia have half such large risk of an event.

Owing to the data basis (retrospective, matched-pairs, low case number), the author is of the opinion that the word "significant" should not be used in this evaluation and analysis with reference to the evaluation of the advantage of also using hyperthermia. However, there are very strong indications that patients benefit from additional local regional hyperthermia.

On, 09/11/2011, a re-analysis of the data of Mr. Mayer, Institute of Epidemiology and Medical Biometry, in co-operation with Prof. Dr. Kron, external employee and lecturer of the Institute of Epidemiology and Medical Biometry, University of Ulm, each at Schwabstr. 13, 89075 Ulm, Director: Prof. Dr. Rainer Muche, took place. The matching concerning nature of the tumour (colon; rectum); tumour stage, type of chemo-immunotherapy) was especially included again in the analysis. From a statistical point of view, it was absolutely necessary to take into account the fact that data of matched-pairs of patients was involved and not data of two independent groups of patients.

The independence can no longer be guaranteed, because it was indeed explicitly provided by means of the three factors "attributes, tumour stage and chemotherapy", that the patients are similar as far as possible in both groups.

The second analysis of progression free survival (PFS), under special consideration of matched-pairs on 9/11/2011 (Benjamin Mayer in co-operation with Dr. Kron, Institute of Epidemiology and Medical Biometry, University of Ulm, Schwabstr. 13, 89075 Ulm, Director: Prof. Dr. Rainer Muche) resulted in the following Kaplan-Meier curve:

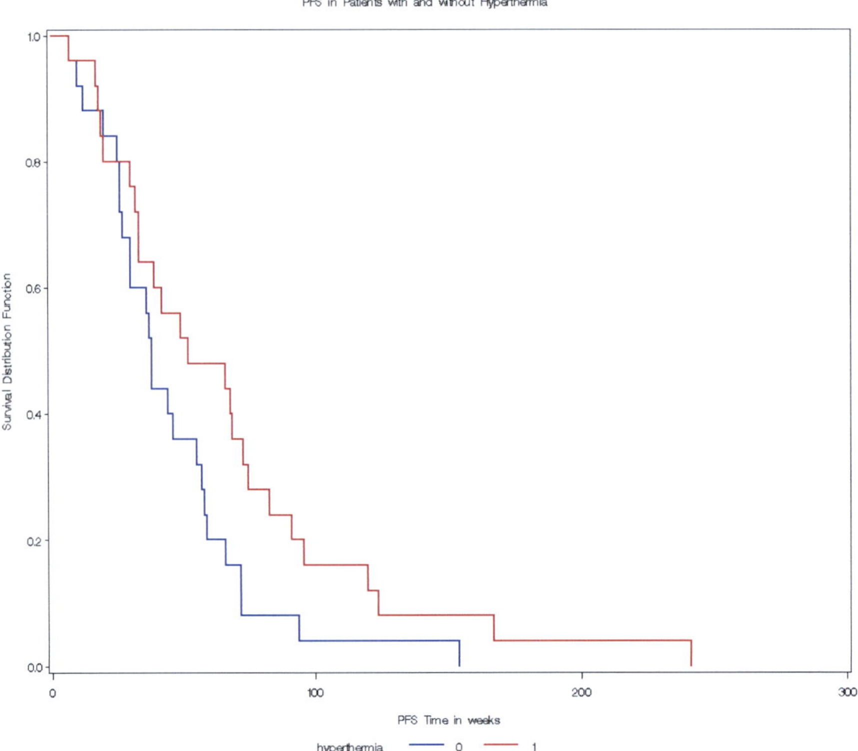

Log-rank test result:
p-value = 0.0633

Result of Cox model for the calculation of HR:
HR = 0.582
95% confidence interval: [0.326,1.042]
p-value = 0.0683

Result of Cox model for the calculation of HR taking into consideration the matching:
HR = 0.733
95% confidence interval: [0.337,1.597]
p-value = 0.4346

The second analysis of overall survival (OS), under special consideration of matched-pairs on 9/11/2011 (Benjamin Mayer in co-operation with Dr. Kron, Institute of Epidemiology and Medical Biometry, University of Ulm, Schwabstr. 13, 89075 Ulm, Director: Prof. Dr. Rainer Muche) resulted in the following Kaplan-Meier curve (see next page):

Log-rank test result:
p-value = 0.0341

Result of Cox model for the calculation of HR:
HR = 0.539
95% confidence interval: [0.299,0.971]
p-value = 0.0397

Result of Cox model for the calculation of HR taking into consideration the matching:
HR = 0.625
95% confidence interval: [0.284,1.377]
p-value = 0.2436

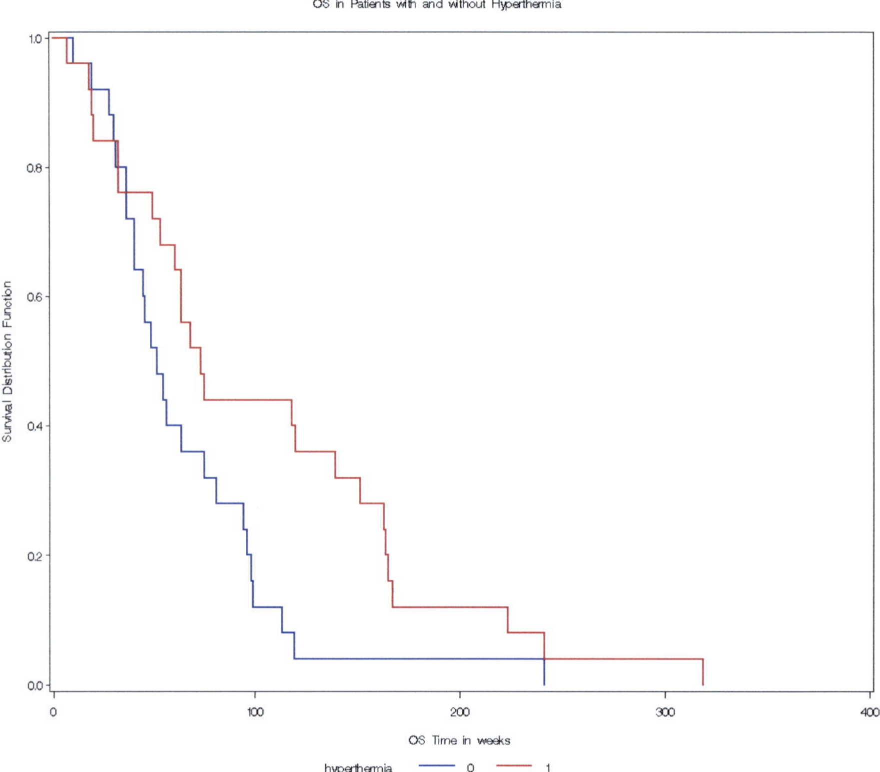

The analysis is interpreted from a statistical point of view and, therefore, finally from the perspective of the author, as follows:

Taking into account the matched-pairs, the HR for PFS and OS are in the second analysis, clearly somewhat less than 1, different from the first analysis and the limits of the respective confidence interval have changed slightly.

However, indeed the interpretation changes especially with regard to the p-values, both of which are no longer significant, and which do not even allow a tendency to be seen, at least for PFS. The reason for these differences is certainly that, under explicit consideration of the matching-structure, the effects within the pairs become more important than would be the case if it were two completely independent groups.

Thus, the two calculated p-values are in contrast to the statement that is read from the log-rank test: this shows an approach to significance in both cases. However, as shown in the unit survival analysis (advanced oncology programme unit 3.1.9), the statements of the log-rank test can no longer be trusted when the curves overlap and overlap again.

In summary, it must be said, therefore, from a statistical point of view that, on the basis of the Cox model, no meaningful differences with respect to hyperthermia therapy for the target variables, PFS and OS, are to be observed.

However, considering not only the statistical analysis, but looking at the two diagrams most pragmatically, one would say from a medical point of view certainly, that hyperthermia patients benefit from treatment to some extent, since the corresponding survival curve for PFS and OS usually lies above the reference curve.

In this respect, a clinical advantage can be assumed even in the absence of statistical significance, and a prospective randomised Phase III study must be waited for until carried out with a relevant case number to finally clarify the clinical use of the method. From the point of view of the signatory, the evidence of a clinical benefit from the present research justifies the initiation of such study.

The following side effects have been observed (cumulative NCI Common Toxicity Criteria, degrees 1-3,[58] in %, multiple entries were possible):

---

[58] NATIONAL CANCER INSTITUTE (2011): ctep.cancer.gov/protocolDevelopment/electronic_applications/ctc.htm

Chemo-immunotherapy:	with hyperthermia	without hyperthermia
Nausea/vomiting	40%	48%
Diarrhoea/gastroenteritis	**32%**	**52%**
Constipation	**16%**	**4%**
Weight loss/loss of appetite/fatigue	20%	20%
Dehydration	4%	0%
Stroke	0%	4%
Dyspnoea	4%	4%
Shivering/fever/ Infections	**32%**	**16%**
Bleeding/nose bleeds/oedema	8%	8%
Vertigo	0%	4%
Polyneuropathy	12%	0%
Pains/ Abdominal pains	4%	4%
Abdominal pains during hyperthermia	8%	0%
Thrombocytopenia	4%	0%
Admission to hospital	0%	0%
Death during treatment	0%	0%
Totals	185%	164%

3/25 patients with no side effects were found in both groups.

Apart from this, side effects tended to increase in the hyperthermia group. In particular, the systemic reaction of “fever”, with its tendency to increase, partly associated with shivering and infections, points to a systemic additional effect of hyperthermia.

In contrast, there is a tendency towards a reduction in diarrhoea and an increase in constipation, possibly attributed to the dehydration effect during hyperthermia, but which was only clinically relevant in one case.

Additional, conceivable side effects (thrombosis and embolism) did not occur,

Severe side effects, especially admission to hospital and death during the study occurred in neither group.

3. Discussion: Integration of Regional Deep Hyperthermia with Oncological Treatment Concepts

The present matched-pair analysis of PFS and OFS yields evidence of an advantage insofar as the effect of systemic cytotoxic first-line treatment can be improved to a significant degree in clinical terms, by means of chemotherapy and antibodies through local regional electro-hyperthermia, for liver metastasis and colorectal carcinoma.

However, the eventual scientific evidence for this thesis can only be proved by means of a multi-centred, double-blind Phase III study with identical chemo-antibody treatment, with and without supplementary hyperthermia.

The performance of this therapy study appears to be difficult to achieve under the current study conditions (absence of therapy standards in palliative first-line systemic treatment with varying combinations of 2-4 cytotoxic substances and possibly 1 or 2 antibodies).

However, this study has been encouraged by me in the appropriate environment (university hospitals with studies in hyperthermia such as Lübeck, Berlin and Munich) and with practising haematologists and oncologists (Federation of practising haematologists and oncologists, abbreviated BNHO) and in oncology organ centres (Colon Centre). Oncologists and experienced radiation therapists are also involved in hyperthermia in these institutions[59], who all want to integrate hyperthermia as an additional pillar of cancer therapy with multimodal concepts.

This applies even more so, because no studies are currently recruiting study patients in Germany regarding colorectal tumours in the metastatic tumour situation or otherwise.

---

[59] Wust, P., Seegenschmidt, H., Burgmoser, G., Feyerabend,T. and M. Molls: *Interdisziplinäre Arbeitsgruppe Hyperthermie. Leitlinien zur Durchführung der loko-regionalen Hyperthermie*, 2001: Krebsgesellschaft.de/download/leitinien_regionale-hyperthermie.pdf

On the other hand, currently intraperitoneal, hyperthermal chemotherapy is being evaluated in Europe for locally advanced colorectal carcinoma with peritoneal carcinoma (Baki Topal, MD, PhD, Leuven, Belgium; Francois Quenet, MD, Va d´Aurelle, France).[60]

4. Summary

Palliative systemic treatment (combinations of cytostatic chemotherapy and antibody therapy) for colorectal carcinomas with liver metastasis has improved the average survival time of patients in the last 20 years of medical development from an average of about 6 to 24 months.[61]

This development has not yet reached its high point with reference to the integration of new drug therapy approaches, in particular as part of the so-called targeted therapy against molecular identifiable approaches.

However, in the course of cancer therapy, the increase in knowledge has continued to develop so that by reason of evasion mechanisms of tumour cells, within the resistance already existing initially, or acquired in the course against cytotoxic drugs, or radiotherapy, the sole approach of a kind of therapy cannot be seen as sufficient. On the contrary, the combined approach of multi-modal therapy concepts involving treatment with and without drugs has been propagated to overcome this primary or secondary resistance. However, a clinical check out of these combinations within randomised-controlled studies of high evidence (Phase III) is only possible under difficult conditions for different reasons (ongoing drug development during recruiting, comorbidity hinders

---

[60] Schlag, P.M. and M. Bamberg: *Rekrutierende Hyperthermiestudien.* – Der Onkologe 11(2010)1095.

[61] Kopetz, S., Chang, G.J. and M.J. Overmann: *Improved survival in metastatic colorectal cancer is associated with adoption of hepatic resection and improved chemotherapy.* – J Clin Oncol 27(2009)3677-83.

a systemic therapy selection for all patients, non-availability of treatment without drugs, no sponsoring by companies that do not manufacture drugs).

However, the counter-argument that the more the better, cannot implicitly be proved with scientific evidence, so that at least, evidence should be aimed for in the Phase II study or in case-control studies.

On the other hand, the uncritical, widely practised use of unproven therapy methods, e.g. the use of local regional thermo-ablation for liver metastases with heat or cold-induced coagulation before the necessary scientific evidence is achieved, is a good example of the intimidating abandonment of a joint scientific basis.

Also the allegation that technical additional methods such as thermo-ablation or hyperthermia are misused commercially can be well understood in the absence of scientific evidence, which can put pressure both on the desire of patients for a successful and well tolerated method of treatment and on doctors. This can be seen for example in postponing the requirement of the treatment targets to be achieved in the development of drugs (to some extent, classification as not-inferior is already sufficient for a standard classification) or the approval owing to a significant advantage in overall survival of a few days (e.g. Tarceva in the case of advanced pancreas carcinoma).

Therefore, in this research, for the preparation of a prospective randomised Phase III study, the advantage regarding the progression free survival and the overall survival of patients with hepatic metastatic colorectal carcinoma by adding local regional deep hyperthermia of the liver for drug systemic treatment was investigated within a case control study (matched-pair analysis) with a total of 25 pairs of patients in 3 practices focusing on oncology in the greater Bonn area.

To this end, the allocation for the case control took place regarding the disease (colon or rectum), the tumour stage (at the time of the first diagnosis) and the type of systemic treatment (chemotherapy or chemo-immunotherapy with antibodies). The addition of the initial stage of the tumour took place for taking into account the biology of the tumour (grading and growth of the tumour at the time of the first diagnosis).

Taking into account the factors for the allocation of the case control (matched-pairs) in the statistics, no results of statistical significance are shown in the final analysis in spite of indications of advantages in PFS and OS in the graphic visual analyses but in the COX models for the calculation of the hazard ratio. The log-rank test cannot be used by reason of the overlapping and re-overlapping curves.

The clinical interpretation of the data with indication of an advantage for the progression free survival and the overall survival represents the basis of an initiation of a prospective, randomised Phase III study for the final test of the question, whether the addition of local regional deep hyperthermia of the liver for liver metastasis of a colorectal carcinoma leads to a significant advantage regarding survival times.

5. Bibliography

ANDREWS, N.W.: *Membrane repair and immunological danger.* – EMBO Rep. 6(2005)826-830.

ANCOCS, G., SZASZ, O. AND A. SZASZ: *Oncothermia treatment of cancer: for the laboratory to clinic.* – Electromagn Biol Med 28(2009)148-165.

ATMACA, A., AL BATRAN, S.E., AND A. NEUMANN: *Whole-body hyperthermia in combination with carboplatin in patients with recurrent ovarian cancer – a Phase II study.* – Gynaecol Cancer 112(2009)384-388.

BAUER, K.D. AND K.J. HENLE: *Arrhenius analysis of heat survival curves form normal and thermotolerant CHO cells.* – Radiat Res 78(1979)251-263.

DAHL, O.: *Interaction of hyperthermia and chemotherapy.* – Recent Results Cancer Res 107(1988)157-169.

COLOMBO, R., DA POZZO, L.F. AND A. SALONIA: *Multicentric study comparing intravesical chemotherapy alone and with local microwave hyperthermia for prophylaxis of recurrence of superficial transitional cell carcinoma.* – J Clin Oncol 21(2003)4270-4276.

DE GRAMONT, A., FIGER, A. AND SEYMOUR, M.: *Leucovorin and fluorouracil with or without oxaliplatin as first-line treatment in advanced colorectal cancer.* – J Clin Oncol 18(2000)2938-47.

DE HAAS-KOCK, D.F., BUIJSEN, J. AND M. PIJLS-JOHANNESMA: *Concomitant hyperthermia and radiation therapy for treating locally advanced rectal cancer.* – Cochrane Database Syst Rev CD006269, 2009.

DEMARIA, S., NG, B. AND M.L. DEVITT: *Ionizing radiation inhibition of distant untreated tumours (abscopal effect) is immune mediated.* – Int J Radiat Oncol Biol Phys 58(2004)862-870.

DEWEY, W.C.: *Arrhenius relationships from the molecule and cell to clinic.* – Int J Hyperthermia 10(2009)457-483.

FOTOPOULOU, C., CHO, C.H. AND R. KRAETSCHELL: *Regional abdominal hyperthermia combined with systemic chemotherapy for the treatment of patients with ovarian cancer relapse: results of a pilot study.* – Int J Hyperthermia 26(2010)118-126.

FRANCKENA, M., STALPERS, L.J. AND P.C. KOPER, P.C.: *Long-term improvement in treatment outcome after radiotherapy and hyperthermia in locoregionally advanced cervix cancer: an update of the Dutch Deep Hyperthermia Trial.* – Int J Radiat Oncol Biol Phys 70(2008)1176-1182.

GELLERMANN, J. AND WUST, P.: *Physikalische und technische Grundlagen der regionalen Tiefenhyperthermie.* – Der Onkologe 16(2010)1052/1053/1054.

GOFRIT, O.N., SHAPIRO, A. AND D. PODE: *Combined local bladder hyperthermia and intravesical chemotherapy for the treatment of high-grade superficial bladder cancer.* –Urology 63(2004)466-471.

HAGER, E.D.: *Deep hyperthermia with radiofrequencies in patients with liver metastases from colorectal cancer.* – Anticancer Res 19(1999)3404-3408.

HAVEMAN, J., RIETBROEK, R.C. AND A. GEERDINK: *Effect of hyperthermia on the cytotoxicity of 2′,2′-difluorodeoxycytidine (gemcitabine) in cultured SW1573cells.* – Int J Cancer 62(1995)627-630.

HIRAOKA, M., JO, S. AND K. AKUTA: *Radiofrequency capacitive hyperthermia for deep-seated tumors* – I. Studies on thermometry. – Cancer 60(1987)121-127.

HOSONO, M., ENDO, K., UEDA, R. AND ONOYAMA, Y.: *Effect of hyperthermia on tumour uptake of radiolabeled anti-neural cell adhesion molecule antibody in small-cell lung cancer xenografts.* – J Nucl Med. 35(1994)504-9.

ISSELS, R.D., LINDNER, L.H. AND J. VERWEIJ: *Neo-adjuvant chemotherapy alone or with regional hyperthermia for locolised high-risk soft-tissue sarcoma: a randomised Phase 3 multicentre study.* – Lancet Oncol 11(2010)561-570.

JONES, E., SECORD, A.A. AND L.R. PROSNITZ: *Intraperitoneal cisplatin and whole adbomen hyperthermia for relapsed ovarian carcinoma.* – Int J Hyperthermia 22(2006)161-172.

KONG, G., BRAUN, R.D. AND M.W. DESWHRIST: *Characterization of the effect of hyperthermia on nanoparticle extravasation from tumour vasculature.* – Cancer Res 61(2001)3027-3032.

KOPETZ, S., CHANG, G.J. AND M.J. OVERMANN: *Improved survival in metastatic colorectal cancer is associated with adoption of hepatic resection and improved chemotherapy.* – J Clin Oncol 27(2009)3677-83.

KONING, G.A., EGGERMONT, A.M. AND L.H. LINDNER: *Hyperthermia and thermosensitive liposomes for improved delivery of chemotherapeutic drugs to solid tumours.* – Pharm Res 27(2010)1750-1754.

LEPOCK, J.R.: *Role of nuclear protein denaturation and aggregation in thermal radiosensitization.* – Int J Hyperthermia 20(2004)115-130.

MATZINGER, P.: *The danger model: A renewed sense of self.* – Science 296(2002)301-305.

MILLER, R.C., ROIZIN-TOWLE, L. AND K. KOMATSU: *Interaction of heat with x-rays and cis-platinum; cell lethality and oncogenic transformation.* – Int J Hyperthermia 5(1989)697-705.

MOLLS, M., VAUPEL, P., NIEDER, C. AND M.S. ANSCHER: *The impact of tumour biology on cancer treatment and multidisciplinary strategies.* – In: BRADY, L.W., HEILMANN, H.P., MOLLS, M. AND J. J. NIEDER (eds.): *Medical radiology.* – Berlin, Heidelberg, New York, 2010, pp 117-128.

MULTHOFF, G. AND U. GAIPL: *Molekulare und immunologische Effekte der Hyperthermie auf Tumorprogression und Metastasierung.* – Der Onkologe 16(2010)1043-1051.

NATIONAL CANCER INSTITUTE (2011): ctep.cancer.gov/protocolDevelopment/electronic_applications/ctc.htm

OTT, J.O., SCHMIDT, M., AND R. SAUER: *Bedeutung der Hyperthermie im Rahmen radioonkologischer Behandlungsstrategien.* – Der Onkologe 16(2010)1072-1078.

OVERGAARD J.: *The current and potential role of hyperthermia in radiotherapy.* – Int J Rad Oncol Biol Phys 16(1989)535-549.

PANAGIOTOU, P., SOSADA, M., SCHERING, S. AND H. KIRCHNER: *Irinotecan plus capecitabine with regional electrohyperthermia of the liver as second line therapy in patients with metastatic colorectal cancer.* – ESHO, Jun 8-11. 2005, Graz, Austria.

Proposed mechanism for the interaction of radiofrequency signals with living matter, demodulation in biological systems. – Workshop, University of Rostock, Germany, 11-13 September 2006.

RIETBROEK, R.C., SCHILTHUIS, M.S. AND P.J.M. BAKKER: *Phase II trial of weekly locoregional hyperthermia and cisplatin in patients with a previously irradiated recurrent carcinoma of the uterine cervix.* – Cancer 79(1997)935-943.

ROMANOWSKI, R., SCHÖTT, C. AND R. ISSELS, R.: *Regionale Hyperthermie mit systemischer Chemotherapie bei Kindern und Jugendlichen: Durchführbarkeit und klinische Verläufe bei 34 intensiv vorbehandelten Patienten mit prognostisch ungünstigen Tumorerkrankungen.* –Klin Padiatr 205(1993)249-256.

ROTI ROTI, J.L.: *Cellular responses to hyperthermia (40-46 degrees C): Cell killing and molecular events.* – Int J Hyperthermia 24(2008)3-15.

SAPARETO, S.A. AND W.C. DEWEY: *Thermal dose determination in cancer therapy.* – Int J Radiat Oncol Biol Phys 10(1984)787-800.

SAVILL, J., DRANSFIELD, I. AND C. GREGORY: *Clearance of apoptotic cells regulates immune responses.* – Nat Rev Immunol 2(2002)965-975.

SCHLAG, P.M. AND M. BAMBERG: *Rekrutierende Hyperthermiestudien.* – Der Onkologe 11(2010)1095.

SHRIVASTAVA, P.K., CALLAHAN, M.K. AND M.M. MAURI: *Treating human cancers with heat shock protein-peptide complexes: The road ahead.* – Expert Opin Biol Ther 9(2009)179-186.

SKITZKI, J.J., REPASKY, E.A. AND S.S. EVANS: *Hyperthermia as an immunotherapy strategy for cancer.* – Curr Opin Invest Drugs 10(2009)550-558.

SONG, C.W., RHEE, J.G. AND C.K. LEE: *Capacitive heating of phantom and human tumors with an 8 MHz radiofrequency applicator (Thermotron RF-8).* – Int J Radiation Oncol Biol Phys 12(1986)365-372.

SZASZ, A., SZASZ, N. AND O. SZASZ, O.: *Oncothermia: Principles and Practices.* – Berlin, Heidelberg, New York, 2011, p.175, Fig. 3.51/p.

468, Appendix 29/pp. 174-242/p.228, Fig. 4.59/p.238, Fig. 4.76/p.239, Fig. 4.78/p.222, Fig. 4.53/p.175, Fig. 4.1.

SZENDRO, P., VINCZE, G. AND A. SZASZ: *Bio Response on white-noise-excitation.* – Electromagn Biol Med 20(2001)215-229.

TOWLE, L.R.: *Hyperthermia and drug resistance.* – In: URANO, M. AND E. DOUBLE (eds.): *Hyperthermia and oncology.* Vol. 4. – Utrecht, 1989, pp. 91-113.

URANO, M., KURODA, M. AND Y. NISHIMURA: *For the clinical application of thermochemotherapy given at mild temperatures.* – Int J Hyperthermia 15(1999)79-107.

VOLL, R.E., HERRMANN, M. AND E.A. ROTH: *Immunosuppressive effects of apoptotic cells.* – Nature 390(1997)350-351.

WESSALOWSKI, R., SCHNEIDER, D.T. AND O. MILS: *An approach for cure: PEI-chemotherapy and regional deep hyperthermia in children and adolescents with unresectable malignant tumors.* – Klin Padiatr 215(2003)303-309.

WITJED, J.A., HENDRICKSEN, K. AND O. GOFRIT: *Intravesical hyperthermia and mitomycin-C for carcinoma in situ of the urinary bladder: experience of the European Synergo® working party.* – World J Urol 27(2009)319-324.

WUST, P., SEEGENSCHMIDT, H., BURGMOSER, G., FEYERABEND,T. AND M. MOLLS: *Interdisziplinäre Arbeitsgruppe Hyperthermie. Leitlinien zur Durchführung der lokoregionalen Hyperthermie,* 2001: Krebsgesellschaft.de/download/leitinien_regionale-hyperthermie.pdf

6. APPENDIX 1.1

Appen-dix	Patients ID	Name	Date of birth	Diagnosis	First diagnosis	Pre-treatment	Kind of Pre-treatment
1	12482	YB	26.06.1946	KolonCa	15.06.2001	Yes	AIO
1,1	11045	SC	21.12.1934	KolonCa	15.02.2005	Yes	AIO
2	81	MJ	06.06.1944	Rectum	22.07.2005	None	None
2,1	8762	PP	01.06.1921	Rectum	18.01.2006	None	None
3	10515	SM	24.08.1967	KolonCa	15.03.2001	Yes	Folfox 4
3,1	6486	TA	21.09.1937	KolonCa	15.12.2004	Yes	AIO
4	9855	SA	07.06.1943	KolonCa	15.04.2006	None	None
4,1	10386	SB	08.09.1941	KolonCa	10.01.2007	None	None
5	8006	SD	04.06.1940	KolonCa	01.01.1998	Yes	AIO
5,1	9041	SA	29.10.1943	KolonCa	15.04.2004	Yes	AIO
6	6344	TK	21.12.1946	KolonCa	10.12.2003	Yes	Folfox 4
6,1	9181	MP	03.10.1937	KolonCa	15.01.2002	Yes	Folfox 4
7	10235	WL	09.05.1930	RectumCa	28.11.2006	Yes	Rectum erlangen
7,1	9789	KM	24.06.1923	RectumCa	15.01.2002	Yes	Rectum erlangen
8	10412	EM	29.05.1969	RectumCa	12.01.2007	None	None
8,1	9934	SW	19.06.1953	RectumCa	15.02.2007	None	None
9	11810	EH	15.09.1943	KolonCa	16.11.2007	None	None
9,1	8160	HPP	17.06.1933	KolonCa	05.08.2005	None	None
10	8732	BE	31.10.1919	KolonCa	29.12.2005	None	None
10,1	7199	MC	14.05.1932	Rectum	10.01.2005	None	None
11	8149	HKH	18.08.1952	KolonCa	05.08.2005	None	None
11,1	11182	RM	24.04.1934	RectumCA	16.07.2007	None	None
12	8085	JB	02.05.1951	KolonCa	22.08.2005	Yes	Folfox 4
12,1	7566	SHJ	29.08.1957	KolonCa	15.12.2004	Yes	AIO
13	11029	KW	03.07.1936	RectumCa	15.05.2007	None	None
13,1	7199	MC	14.05.1932	RectumCa	12.04.2004	None	None
14	8508	KG	30.09.1940	KolonCa	15.03.2005	None	None
14,1	9829	KHJ	13.09.1958	KolonCa	26.08.2005	None	None
15	8216	LPD	29.08.1939	KolonCa	20.01.2004	Yes	AIO
15,1	10877	PJ	09.07.1932	KolonCa	03.01.2005	Yes	AIO
16	10138	OE	03.03.1926	RectumCa	17.10.2006	None	None
16,1	8541	HG	15.04.1926	RectumCa	27.10.2005	None	None
17	8822	WJ	01.10.1941	KolonCa	10.01.2006	None	None
17,1	8309	EG	07.02.1942	KolonCa	16.09.2005	None	None
18	15631	NKH	13.05.1931	KolonCa	09.02.2007	None	None
18,1	12654	GU	13.03.1939	KolonCa	16.02.2005	Yes	Folfox 4
19	16609	PJ	21.03.1945	KolonCa	17.06.2010	None	None
19,1	11111	GG	24.09.1936	KolonCa	13.02.2009	None	None
20	17445	PH	11.08.1957	KolonCa	27.10.2010	None	None
20,1	13276	MI	09.12.1942	KolonCa	28.08.2008	None	None
21	16786	QHD	30.01.1937	KolonCa	15.05.2010	None	None
21,1	9224	LT	28.11.1931	KolonCa	03.04.2006	None	None
22	13488	SHJ	01.02.1936	RectumCa	01.01.2002	Yes	Rectum erlangen
22,1	7695	RC	30.03.1928	RectumCa	11.03.2005	Yes	Rectum erlangen
23	18630	SR	16.11.1954	KolonCa	20.06.2011	None	None
23,1	9454	SJ	04.12.1939	KolonCa	29.05.2006	None	None
24	14456	TG	15.11.1942	KolonCa	10.09.2009	None	None
24,1	8580	SR	14.06.1931	KolonCa	21.11.2005	None	None
25	14346	WG	05.05.1938	RectumCa	01.01.1998	None	None
25,1	8541	HG	05.04.1926	RectumCa	01.06.2002	None	None

6. APPENDIX 1.2

Appen-dix	TNM	Metastasis diagnosis	Metastasis localisation	Chemotherapy regime	H=Hyperthermia
1	T3 NO MO G2	06.03.2008	HEP	Folfox 4	
1,1	T3 NO MO G2	11.06.2007	HEP	Folfox 4	0
2	T4 N1 M1 G2	22.07.2005	HEP	AIO	H
2,1	T4 N1 M1 G2	18.01.2006	HEP	AIO	0
3	T4 N2 M0 G2	05.02.2007	HEP	Bevacizumab Irinotecan AIO	H
3,1	T4 N2 M0 G2	03.05.2007	HEP	Bevacizumab Irinotecan AIO	0
4	T3 N2 M1 G3	15.04.2006	HEP	Bevacizumab Irinotecan AIO	H
4,1	T3 N2 M1 G3	10.01.2007	HEP	Bevacizumab Irinotecan AIO	0
5	T3 N0 M0 G2	23.06.2005	HEP	Bevacizumab Irinotecan AIO	H
5,1	T3 N0 M0 G2	15.02.2006	HEP	Bevacizumab Irinotecan AIO	0
6	T3 N0 M0 G2	22.01.2007	HEP	AIO	H
6,1	T3 N0 M0 G2	07.04.2006	HEP	AIO	0
7	T2 N1 M0 G3	25.07.2007	HEP, PUL	Bevacizumab AIO	H
7,1	T3 N1 M0 G3	29.08.2006	HEP, PUL	Bevacizumab AIO	0
8	T3 N2 M1 G3	12.01.2007	HEP	Bevacizumab Irinotecan AIO	H
8,1	T3 N2 M1 G3	15.02.2007	HEP	Bevacizumab Irinotecan AIO	0
9	T3 N1 M1 G3	16.11.2007	HEP	Bevacizumab Irinotecan AIO	H
9,1	T3 N1 M1 G3	05.08.2005	HEP	Bevacizumab Irinotecan AIO	0
10	T3 N2 M1 G3	29.12.2005	HEP	Bevacizumab AIO	H
10,1	T3 N2 M1 G3	10.01.2005	HEP	Bevacizumab AIO	0
11	T4 N0 M1 G2	05.08.2005	HEP, PUL	Bevacizumab Irinotecan AIO	H
11,1	T4 N0 M1 G2	16.07.2007	HEP, PUL	Bevacizumab Irinotecan AIO	0
12	T4 N2 M0 G3	11.01.2006	HEP	Bevacizumab Irinotecan AIO	H
12,1	T4 N2 M0 G3	07.09.2007	HEP	Bevacizumab Irinotecan AIO	0
13	T3 N2 M1 G3	15.05.2007	HEP	Folfox 4	H
13,1	T3 N2 M1 G3	12.04.2004	HEP	Folfox 4	0
14	T3 N1 M1 G2	15.03.2005	HEP	Bevacizumab Irinotecan AIO	H
14,1	T3 N1 M1 G2	24.08.2006	HEP	Bevacizumab Irinotecan AIO	0
15	T3 N2 M0 G3	06.03.2006	HEP	MitoXeloda	H
15,1	T3 N2 M0 G3	12.04.2007	HEP	MitoXeloda	0
16	T4 N2 M1 G3	17.10.2006	HEP	Bevacizumab AIO	H
16,1	T4 N2 M1 G3	27.10.2005	HEP	Bevacizumab AIO	0
17	T2 N1 M1 G3	10.01.2006	HEP	Bevacizumab Irinotecan AIO	H
17,1	T3 N1 M1 G3	16.09.2005	HEP	Bevacizumab Irinotecan AIO	0
18	T3 N2 M0 G3	06.11.2009	HEP	BevacizumabXelodaoxaliplatin	H
18,1	T3 N1 M0 G3	14.04.2008	HEP	BevacizumabXelodaoxaliplatin	0
19	T3 N2 M1 G2	17.06.2010	HEP	Folfox 4	H
19,1	T3 N2 M1 G2	13.02.2009	HEP	Folfox 4	0
20	T2 N1 M1 G2	27.10.2010	HEP	Folfox 4	H
20,1	T2 N1 M1 G2	28.08.2008	HEP	Folfox 6	0
21	T3 N1 M1 G3	15.05.2010	HEP	AIO	H
21,1	T3 N1 M1 G3	03.04.2006	HEP	AIO	0
22	T3 N0 M0 G2	01.01.2005	HEP	AIO	H
22,1	T3 N0 M0 G2	15.08.2008	HEP	AIO	0
23	T3 N1 M1 G3	20.06.2011	HEP	Folfox 4	H
23,1	T3 N1 M1 G3	29.05.2006	HEP	Folfox 4	0
24	T3 N2 M1 G2	10.06.2009	HEP	Bevacizumab Irinotecan AIO	H
24,1	T3 N2 M1 G2	21.11.2005	HEP	Bevacizumab Irinotecan AIO	0
25	T2 N0 M0 G2	27.03.2009	HEP	BevacizumabFolFOX4	H
25,1	T2 N0 M0 G2	29.11.2006	HEP	BevacizumabFolFOX4	0

6. APPENDIX 1.3

Appen-dix	Number of hyperthermia	Best- response	PFS in Weeks	OS in Weeks	Comment
1	6	CR	75	75	Lost of follow up
1,1	0	PR	26	36	
2	12	CR	69	163	
2,1	0	PR	94	113	
3	20	PR	91	163	
3,1	0	PR	59	81	
4	22	PR	120	120	
4,1	0	PR	30	30	
5	34	CR	124	319	alive
5,1	0	PR	38	56	
6	12	CR	241	241	alive
6,1	0	PR	25	28	Lost of follow up
7	16	PR	39	118	
7,1	0	PR	26	48	
8	31	PR	96	223	
8,1	0	CR	154	241	alive
9	6	PR	20	32	
9,1	0	PR	30	40	
10	3	SD	17	20	
10,1	0	PR	72	119	
11	17	PR	52	139	
11,1	0	SD	10	10	
12	2	SD	7	7	
12,1	0	PR	72	98	
13	4	PR	30	32	
13,1	0	PR	38	94	
14	17	PR	66	151	
14,1	0	PR	66	96	
15	16	PR	32	63	
15,1	0	SD	27	40	
16	22	PR	42	63	
16,1	0	PR	55	63	Lost of follow up
17	18	PR	19	19	
17,1	0	PR	44	44	
18	54	PR	167	167	
18,1	0	PR	36	36	
19	26	CR	68	68	alive
19,1	0		58	75	
20	12	CR	49	49	alive
20,1	0	PR	20	45	Lost of follow up
21	32	PR	73	73	alive
21,1	0	PR	57	99	
22	24	PR	83	165	
22,1	0	SD	12	19	
23	8	PR	18	18	alive
23,1	0	PR	46	54	
24	12	PR	33	53	
24,1	0	PR	37	51	
25	8	PR	33	60	
25,1	0	PR	7	31	Comment

6. Appendix 1.4

Appen-dix	Side effects NCI 1-3
1	Hand-Food-Syndrom
1,1	Diarrhoea
2	Nausea
2,1	Vomiting, Nausea, Apoplexia, Diarrhoea
3	Gastroenteritis, Fever, Weight Loss
3,1	Fever, Diarrhoea, Chills
4	Exsiccosis
4,1	Anorexia
5	Diarrhoea, Vomiting
5,1	Nausea, Diarrhoe, Edema
6	Chills, Port infection, Bleeding with Phenprocoumon
6,1	Vertigo, Nausea, Diarrhoea
7	Diarrhea, Gastric ulcer, Abdominal pain
7,1	Nausea, Diarrhoe, Edema
8	Diarrhoea
8,1	Enteritis, Diarrhoea
9	Dyspnoa
9,1	Oral Mucositis, Fever, Chills
10	Pain during Hyperthermia
10,1	Cramps after Chemotherapy
11	Flue symptoms, Polyneuropathy
11,1	None
12	Thrombocytopenia
12,1	Nausea, Vomiting
13	Anorexia, Weight loss
13,1	Nausea
14	Constipation, Urinary tract infection
14,1	Diarrhoea
15	None
15,1	Weight loss
16	Anorexia, Constipation, Nausea, Diarrhoea, Fever
16,1	None
17	Constipation, Diarrhoea, Fever
17,1	Nausea, Diarrhoea, Weight loss,
18	Diarrhoea, Weight loss
18,1	Diarrhoea
19	Polyneuropathy
19,1	Fatigue
20	None
20,1	Nause, Vomiting
21	Abdominal pain during Hyperthermia, Nausea, Vomiting
21,1	Diarrhoea
22	None
22,1	Nausea, Weight Loss
23	Polyneuropathy, Dysgeusia
23,1	Diarrhoea, Abdominal pain in the lower abdomen
24	Constipation, Epistaxis, Fever, Nausea
24,1	Diarrhoea, Constipation
25	Diarrhoea, Nausea
25,1	None

	PFS	OS
With H	66,55	104,02
Without H	41,83	60,38
Advantage in %	0,37	0,42